Grief Diaries

SURVIVING LOSS BY SUICIDE

12 True stories about
surviving the aftermath of
losing a loved one to suicide

LYNDA CHELDELIN FELL

WITH

SHARON EHLERS

FOREWORD BY EMILY BARNHARDT

A portion of proceeds from the sale of this book is
donated to American Foundation for Suicide Prevention,
the nation's largest nonprofit dedicated to saving
lives and bringing hope to those affected by suicide.
For more information, visit https://afsp.org.

Grief Diaries
Surviving Loss by Suicide – 1st ed.
True stories about surviving loss by suicide.
Lynda Cheldelin Fell/Sharon Ehlers
Grief Diaries www.GriefDiaries.com

Cover Design by AlyBlue Media, LLC
Interior Design by AlyBlue Media LLC
Published by AlyBlue Media, LLC

ISBN: 978-1-944328-03-0
Library of Congress Control Number: 2015916891
AlyBlue Media, LLC
Ferndale, WA 98248
www.AlyBlueMedia.com

PRINTED IN THE UNITED STATES OF AMERICA

GRIEF DIARIES

TESTIMONIALS

"CRITICALLY IMPORTANT . . . I want to say to Lynda that what you are doing is so critically important." –DR. BERNICE A. KING, Daughter of Dr. Martin Luther King

"INSPIRATIONAL . . . Grief Diaries is the result of heartfelt testimonials from a dedicated and loving group of people. By sharing their stories, the reader will find inspiration and a renewed sense of comfort as they move through their own journey." -CANDACE LIGHTNER, Founder of Mothers Against Drunk Driving

"DEEPLY INTIMATE . . . Grief Diaries is a deeply intimate, authentic collection of narratives that speak to the powerful, often ambiguous, and wide spectrum of emotions that arise from loss." -DR. ERICA GOLDBLATT HYATT, Chair of Psychology, Bryn Athyn College

"BRAVE . . . The brave individuals who share their truth in this book do it for the benefit of all." CAROLYN COSTIN - Founder, Monte Nido Treatment Centers

"VITAL . . . Grief Diaries: Surviving Loss of a Pregnancy gives voice to the thousands of women who face this painful journey every day. Often alone in their time of need, these stories will play a vital role in surrounding each reader with warmth and comfort as they seek understanding and healing in the aftermath of their own loss." -JENNIFER CLARKE, obstetrical R.N., Perinatal Bereavement Committee at AMITA Health Adventist Medical Center

"HOPE AND HEALING . . . You are a pioneer in this field and you are breaking the trail for others to find hope and healing." -KRISTI SMITH, Bestselling Author & International Speaker

"A FORCE . . .The writers of this project, the Grief Diaries anthology series, are a force to be reckoned with. I'm betting we will be agents of great change." -MARY LEE ROBINSON, Author and Founder of Set an Extra Plate initiative

"MOVING . . . In Grief Diaries, the stories are not only moving but often provide a rich background for any mourner to find a gem of insight that can be used in coping with loss. Reread each story with pen in hand and you will find many that are just right for you." -DR. LOUIS LAGRAND, Author of Healing Grief, Finding Peace

"HEALING . . . Grief Diaries gives voice to a grief so private, most women bear it alone. These diaries can heal hearts and begin to build community and acceptance to speak the unspeakable. Share this book with your sisters, mothers, grandmothers and friends who have faced grief. Pour a cup of tea together and know that you are no longer alone." -DIANNA VAGIANOS ARMENTROUT, Poetry Therapist & Author of Walking the Labyrinth of My Heart: A Journey of Pregnancy, Grief and Infant Death

"STUNNING . . . Grief Diaries treats the reader to a rare combination of candor and fragility through the eyes of the bereaved. Delving into the deepest recesses of the heartbroken, the reader easily identifies with the diverse collection of stories and richly colored threads of profound love that create a stunning read full of comfort and hope." -DR. GLORIA HORSLEY, President, Open to Hope Foundation

"WONDERFUL . . .Grief Diaries is a wonderful computation of stories written by the best of experts, the bereaved themselves. Thank you for building awareness about a topic so near and dear to my heart." -DR. HEIDI HORSLEY, Adjunct Professor, School of Social Work, Columbia University, Author, Co-Founder of Open to Hope Organization

"GLOBAL . . .One of The Five Facets of Healing mantras is together we can heal a world of hurt. This anthology series is testimony to the power we have as global neighbors to do just that." -ANNAH ELIZABETH, Founder of The Five Facets of Healing

DEDICATION

To our beloved:
Moments are fleeting,
memories are permanent,
love is forever.

Timothy John Cole
Hannah Elizabeth Flanery
Joy Ruth Frownfelter
Brian Andrew Habedank
William Hayes Holesapple
James Cameron Mjelve
Austin Jon Park
John Kirby Reilly
Elizabeth Noel Sclafani

CONTENTS

BY EMILY BARNHARDT

FOREWORD

To the brave hearts reading this book,

The loss of my roommate and my close friend to suicide is the hardest thing I've ever faced. It's been a devastating experience beyond description. I've cried countless heart-wrenching tears while facing questions with no answers. I've wrestled with isolation and confusion over how to face the myriad opinions, judgments, and perspectives on suicide. I've observed the common misunderstandings about suicide loss and bereavement. But through it all, I've learned many truths. I've learned that the bereaved are often handed a variety of well-intentioned grief-tutorials from others. Each tutorial suggests different answers to the age-old question marks of grief, such as its timeframe, the best approach to grieving, and which milestones indicate progress. I've also learned that the correct answer to those numerous question marks of grief is that there is no definitive answer – not a universal one, at least.

My personal experience has led me to see just how imperative it is for our world to better understand loss by suicide, and how each loss is unique. As a survivor of suicide loss, I still cannot fully understand the journey of another suicide loss survivor. Our journeys are different, our personalities are different, and the circumstances of our losses are different. These differences, in addition to differences in cultural and religious beliefs, will diversify how each of us process such a trauma.

Available resources that truthfully articulate our parallel yet distinctive journeys are scarce. So we've created one, and you're holding it in your hands right now. This book is a resource that provides deeply emotional and personal insights that expand beyond the boundaries of simple research, statistics, and facts about grief. The pages of this book are filled with raw, candid, and deeply authentic voices from all walks of life, coming together to share our experience. Each story, tearfully and painstakingly penned, expands our awareness of the unique journey one faces in the wake of losing a loved one by suicide.

To readers who are grieving a loss by suicide:

This book is designed to offer you a sense of comfort and relief in knowing you aren't alone. While we hate having you join our ranks, we welcome you with open arms. As you read the collection of stories, we hope you feel us walking alongside you. Our hope is that our words will provide a sense of with-ness to those who feel alone, offer validation to those who feel misunderstood, share hope to those feeling hopeless, and present understanding when none seems possible. As you adjust and walk through your loss, you will step forward, backwards, sideways, and diagonally. Grief often feels disorienting and directionless, but you will find your way again, however long it takes. Your story, my friend, is not over. If our stories ended when our loved one passed, we wouldn't be here writing and sharing our journeys with you. We know what it's like to feel lost, to wrestle with the unanswerable questions, the memories, and the haunting images. We understand that broken videotape that plays in your head, the one where you retrace your steps and question all the moments leading up to the unimaginable. We're sharing our stories because we want you to know you aren't alone; and we hope that any insight we share might help you.

To readers who haven't lost a loved one to suicide:

Thank you. Thank you for opening this book; you are a gift to us. Whether you're a friend or family member looking to support the bereaved, whether you work in the mental health field, volunteer or work with a bereaved community, or whether you read this book simply out of curiosity, you will find valuable insight and awareness toward the experience of suicide loss survivors. I want to thank you for your willingness and desire to step inside a world with no answers. I honor you and thank you for reading these stories and wanting to gain more awareness about suicide. You never know, one day you may save a life.

Sharing a loss like this binds us together in a way few things can. We are sharing our diverse stories for one unified purpose – to help others and to be a voice. We each bring our own flame of experience to this book. When combined, our flames unite and burn brighter, like a beacon for others in need.

Surviving loss by suicide requires a village of support. And you've found such a village. Although each journey is unique, when combined, they form a collection offering hope that this journey is survivable. Each of the writers contained within are living proof. There is also hope beyond merely surviving the journey. We can find purpose that enables us to thrive again.

Wishing comfort and validation to those grieving, and insight and passion to those wanting to understand,

EMILY BARNHARDT

BY LYNDA CHELDELIN FELL

PREFACE

One night in 2007, I had one of *those* dreams, the vivid kind you can't shake. In the dream, I was the front seat passenger in a car and my daughter Aly was sitting behind the driver. Suddenly, the car missed a curve in the road and sailed into a lake. The driver and I escaped the sinking car, but Aly did not. My beloved daughter was gone. The only evidence left behind was a book floating in the water where she disappeared.

Two years later, on August 5, 2009, that horrible nightmare became reality when Aly died as a back seat passenger in a car accident. Returning home from a swim meet, the car carrying Aly and two of her teammates was T-boned by a father coming home from work. My beautiful fifteen-year-old daughter took the brunt of the impact, and died instantly. She was the only fatality.

Just when I thought life couldn't get any worse, it did. My dear sweet hubby buried his head—and grief—in the sand. He escaped into eighty-hour work weeks, more wine, more food, and less talking. His blood pressure shot up, his cholesterol went off the chart, and the perfect storm arrived on June 4, 2012. In an instant, my husband felt a strange warmth spread inside his head. He began drooling, and couldn't speak. My 46-years-young soulmate was having a major stroke.

My husband survived the stroke, but couldn't speak, read, or write, and his right side was paralyzed. He needed assistance just to sit up in bed. He needed full-time care. Still reeling from the loss of our daughter, I found myself again thrust into a fog of grief so thick, I couldn't see through the storm. Adrenaline and autopilot resumed their familiar place at the helm.

In the aftermath of losing Aly and my husband's stroke, I eventually discovered that helping others was a powerful way to heal my own heart. The Grief Diaries series was born and built on this belief. By writing books narrating our journeys, our written words become a portable support group for others. When we swap stories, we feel less alone. It is comforting to know someone else understands the shoes we walk in, and the challenges we face along the way. Which brings us to this book, *Grief Diaries: Surviving Loss by Suicide*. Losing a loved one to such a senseless act can steal your soul and leave you with more questions than answers. Further, you might encounter people who don't understand your emotions or, worse, lack compassion for your journey. This is where the Grief Diaries series can help.

Helen Keller once said, "Walking with a friend in the dark is better than walking alone in the light." This is especially true in the aftermath of a life-changing experience. If you've lost a loved one to suicide, the following true stories are written by courageous people who know exactly how you feel, for they've been in your shoes and walked the same path. Perhaps the shoes are a different size or style, but I hope you find comfort in these stories and the understanding that you aren't truly alone. For we walk ahead, behind, and right beside you.

Wishing you healing, and hope from the Grief Diaries village.

Warm regards,

Lynda Cheldelin Fell

Creator, Grief Diaries

CHAPTER ONE

THE BEGINNING

> Tears have a wisdom all their own. They come when a person has relaxed enough to let go and to work through his sorrow. They are the natural bleeding of an emotional wound, carrying the poison out of the system. Here lies the road to recovery. -F. ALEXANDER MAGOUN

Grief and sorrow are as unique to each individual as his or her fingerprints. To fully appreciate one's perspective, it is helpful to understand one's journey. In this chapter each writer shares that moment when they lost their loved one to suicide to help you understand when life as they knew it ended, and a new one began.

*

KAYLA ARNOLD

Kayla's uncle Tim

died in 2001 at age 34

My uncle and aunt had gotten into an argument. It was such a minor argument, but my uncle told my aunt to leave. He had the gun in his hand, and when my aunt went into the backyard and called 911, while she was on the phone with dispatchers my uncle put the gun to his head and pulled the trigger.

They lived in a very little town named Homer. So when the gunshot happened while my aunt was on the phone with dispatchers, they tried to make it to my uncle as quickly as they could. When they got there only minutes later, it was too late. The single gunshot killed him instantly. There wasn't even an ounce of hope; he was gone in a matter of seconds. His precious, valuable life was gone!

That is the story of how it happened, but here is what I relive over and over again. I was twelve years old. I came downstairs to go to the bathroom. I saw my mom on the phone and she seemed really upset. She told me to go back to bed, that everything was okay. I felt uneasy about it, but did as she asked. A little while later I woke up and needed to go to the bathroom again. So I walked downstairs only to find my grandma sitting in the living room watching TV. She told me to come sit with her. I remember thinking that this was very odd because it was a school night, but I sat next to her and together we watched the first ever finale of Survivor. And then the phone rang. I never would have guessed that phone call would forever change my life.

I remember my grandma answering, and it was my dad calling. He asked Grandma if anyone had awakened. My grandma said I was awake, and he asked to talk to me. I took the phone from my grandma and my dad asked me how I was. I said I was okay. He said, "I have some bad news, honey." At this point I didn't know what to think. I heard the sadness in my dad's voice and I heard his voice crack a little bit. He said, "Honey, I'm sorry, but Uncle Tim is not with us anymore."

I remember being so confused and in shock. What did he mean? Tears were streaming down my face. My dad said, "Uncle Tim died tonight, baby. I am SO sorry!" And at this point all I remember is crying; I couldn't do anything but cry! My grandma hugged me and I sat there crying with her until my parents got home. And then I cried with them.

When my parents arrived home, they explained to me that my uncle had killed himself, that he took his gun and shot himself in the head. They did everything they could to try to calm me down, because I was so upset! I lay on the couch to try to sleep the rest of the night, because I didn't want to wake my sisters up if I cried in the bedroom. When morning came and my sisters woke up, my world shattered a little more as they were told the painful news. I watched their hearts shatter just like mine had just hours before! I saw the same confusion and shock that I was feeling! I felt horrible, because I didn't know how to make it better for them when I couldn't even make it better for myself!

On May 3, 2001, we lost one of the most important people in our lives. I can honestly say that our lives have never been the same.

*

EMILY BARNHARDT
Emily's friend and roommate Hannah
died in 2014 at age 20

There is a certain type of person who, when he or she walks into a room, the atmosphere changes. It suddenly becomes more vibrant and exciting. It's the type of person you know you can count on - the type of person who makes you feel deeply loved, and the type of person whose energy and laugh are contagious. That was Hannah.

She was one of my best friends and also my roommate. We met each other in south Florida and quickly connected, so moving into an apartment together was the perfect fit. Everyone's initial response to seeing a picture of Hannah was how beautiful she was. She was incredibly beautiful, yes, but the most beautiful thing about her was her heart. She lived passionately, loved deeply and had a lively spirit. We always had fun together, and I have precious memories of our many spontaneous adventures.

The deep authenticity in our friendship was what meant the most to me. We did life together. Neither of us had any family in Florida, so we were each other's family. Hannah was a truly loyal and supportive friend and made me feel so important and loved. She embodied confidence and joy.

What most people didn't know, however, was how much Hannah struggled with insecurity over her potential, her personality, her worth, her relationships and her future. I never understood why she felt so self-conscious; she was such a lovable, smart, fun and valuable girl. I'll never be able to understand exactly how it felt to be in her head, but from talks we had, I knew Hannah was struggling to feel hopeful about her ability to overcome the internal battles in her mind and to succeed at all the dreams she had for her life. Hannah had been going through a particularly rough patch when she took her life. Her insecurities were affecting her relationships, she doubted her potential in pursuing a career in nursing, and she felt stressed out handling the responsibilities of life on top of her emotional battles.

A few days before her death, Hannah came home crying and told me she had been fired from the job she loved. Other events of that weekend had been extremely tough as well. On the evening of May 5, I was sitting at a restaurant when I got a call from her mother, who lives in a different state. She was concerned about Hannah's well-being and asked if I had talked to Hannah that day. I hadn't been home and hadn't talked to her, so when I got off the phone with her mom, I called her. Hannah was crying and obviously in distress when she answered, so I told her I would meet up with her and help her figure out how to get through whatever was going on. I needed to close my check at the restaurant, so I told Hannah I would call her right back to figure out where we should meet. But when I called back shortly after, she didn't answer. You know that bad gut feeling you sometimes get in a certain situation? I felt that, so I went looking for her. I drove around for hours, looking everywhere I could think of where Hannah might be, but had no luck. When it got late and I ran out of ideas, I finally had to return to our apartment for the night. I hoped maybe Hannah had fallen asleep at a coworker's house or somewhere similar.

The next morning, her mother called me at 8 a.m. to tell me that Hannah had taken her life that night. It happened shortly after I'd spoken to her. She was at her boyfriend's apartment and was found that night by his roommate. The police contacted Hannah's parents in Tennessee shortly after. I'll never forget that phone call from her mother. I'll never forget the way my phone slipped out of my hand as I leaned on a chair for support, shaking and struggling to breathe. My thoughts were racing, yet the only thought that was clear was, "This isn't real. This can't be happening." I remember laying on the floor at one point, because the solidity of the floor was the only sense of stability I could find in that moment. I remember the gut-wrenching sobs, sometimes so deep that there were moments no sound even came out of my mouth.

Losing someone to suicide forever alters your life and who you are. Hannah's death has changed my perspective on life, my priorities, my relationships, my routine, and my heart. Some changes are good, while some have felt damaging. I have hope that the changes that currently feel negative will be redeemed and healed as my journey continues. Because Hannah was part of my daily life and one of my best friends, I think I took too many moments with her for granted, because I assumed we had a lifetime of moments ahead of us. I didn't realize just how deeply my life was intertwined with hers until she was ripped away from it, and I found myself left with the sharp, jagged edges around a crater where her presence once was.

I was forced to start a new chapter in life, even though I hadn't finished writing the one before. I've stood on wobbly feet the past year, looking at a new chapter I wasn't prepared for and didn't want, trying to figure out exactly how it has changed me and how to find solid ground again. I've grappled with the concept of "closure" and wondered if it's even possible.

Experiencing this level of grief itself has changed me forever. I've learned that grief isn't a coat you put on and then take off once you feel warm again. In a way, you have to absorb grief. It's been a process of acceptance and a process of change and adjustment for me. It has become a part of me, not in the sense that it is my identity, but in the sense that it has redefined the person I am.

I ask myself exactly how Hannah's death has changed me, but I honestly don't think I fully know yet. I know that time will reveal more, but for now there are a few things I do know. I know that since Hannah died, I have a deeper level of compassion, love, and concern over the well-being of others than I ever did before. I've become more sensitive and educated in how to support people in ways that will be most helpful to them. I've found a deep desire to make a difference, to stand up for those who suffer silently and could too easily slip under the radar. I've found a voice to advocate for those who suffer from mental illness. I want to be a light in the darkness. And although Hannah's death itself will never be something I view as "good," I do know that the qualities I've gained are good gifts, because they make me a stronger, more loving and more dependable person. And I am grateful for that.

*

CHRISTINE BASTONE
Christine's sister Elizabeth
died in 2012 at age 38

I think that my sister, whom we called Liz, was troubled for most, if not all, of her life. From the toddler who carried around that pillow that she had to have...to the young lady who pulled her hair out...to the woman who couldn't change her negative thinking no matter how hard she tried. I know there are some people who probably think that Liz did not try to change her negative thinking...but as we talked about it once, I can tell you that she did. Believe me, I can identify with that. I too suffer from it, although to a lesser extent, and have tried to change it myself.

I believe that what my sister Pam said in Liz's eulogy is right: that Liz had a vision in her mind of what life was supposed to be like, and what people were supposed to be like. And I also think that she just couldn't figure out a way to accept that both life and people were not like they were in that vision. In addition, I think Liz was more of a perfectionist than any of us ever knew. She certainly came by her perfectionist tendencies honestly, as she comes from a whole family of them! She was also very sensitive. In her own words, "I tend to take things very seriously, because I am too sensitive for my own good. I always take things to heart." Being sensitive is both good and bad...a strength and a weakness. I should know; I'm very sensitive too.

About two years before her death, Liz and I had a conversation on MySpace about men. She was extremely negative about them. I think she went through more than any of us ever knew with some of them. Now I wish I had paid a little more attention to the surveys she posted as MySpace bulletins. Because in one of them, Liz was asked, "Have you ever been hit by the opposite sex?" And she said, "Yep." I find myself wanting to know who the creep was who did that! I also find myself wanting to know how many times it happened. I really, really hope it was a one-time thing. But, before she died, I had absolutely no idea that she had ever suffered actual physical abuse from anyone.

Liz was not known for being a forgiving person. But I think the reason that she couldn't forgive was that she couldn't forget. Whatever the things were that had happened, I think they would be right in front of her face all the time, and she just couldn't let it go. There's no denying that Liz was difficult. Normally it takes two people to fight, but not with her. She would follow you around the house talking about whatever it was that she was upset about until you couldn't take it anymore, and you yelled at her.

Liz had some sort of physical problem that for years she and her husband tried to figure out what it was, and what to do about it. She even thought they had figured it out a few times. This was especially true in 2009. When I saw her that December, she said she had a major vitamin D deficiency. But she had been taking a prescription strength dose of it for a while, and she was obviously doing great.

Less than two years later Liz was very unhappy in her marriage, and wanted a divorce. We found this out during a Thanksgiving vacation that she took a little over two months before she died. This vacation was a disaster as Liz fought with both her husband and her parents. I don't know of any other event between then and the day she died that led to her suicide.

On Friday, February 10, 2012, Liz's husband came home and found her already dead. I did not find out until the next evening. My father didn't want my mother to call me until he got back from being out of town. And so it came to be a little past 8:00 pm on February 11, that my father, along with my mother, called me to tell me the shocking news.

My sister's death has changed my life. It has made me a little more outspoken. It caused me to question everything I was ever taught to believe, and has changed those beliefs a little. It has made me extremely sensitive to the way we talk about suicide, and how it is portrayed on TV shows and in the movies.

Overall, I think that it has made me a more tolerant person. And yet, in a way, it has also made me less tolerant too. I say that because now I have absolutely no patience with people who are mean, unkind or cruel. And last, but certainly not least, it has brought a lot of great people into my life whom I have gotten to know through the online grief support groups that I have joined.

*

SHARON EHLERS
Sharon's best friend Joy died in 2009 at age 52
Sharon's former fiancé John died in 2012 at age 59

I met my best friend, Joy, when we were working together back in the late 1980s. She was just like her name: vivacious, happy and joyful. With her bright blonde hair, she lit up any room she walked into. Joy had Tourette's syndrome, but it never stopped her from being who she was meant to be. She smoked, she drank, and told the best "blonde" jokes around. She made everyone around her feel at ease.

In the early 1990s we evolved from being coworkers into being great friends. Joy was one of the most thoughtful people I knew. As we spent more time together and became closer friends, I noticed that there was also a lot of pain in Joy's life. When she was going through a particularly difficult time with her husband, I got that "first call" when I was at work. She told me she had taken some pills and couldn't stay awake. I left my office and rushed to her house. That was my first experience with anyone not wanting to live. I remember urging her to talk to a therapist and to her husband about what she was feeling. She did, and things got better.

Over the course of the next ten to fifteen years, Joy was on a rollercoaster of emotions. Her husband decided they would retire (he was ten years older than Joy, who was not even close to retirement age) and move to Las Vegas. Joy was devastated. Her job, family and friends were all in California. She had no desire to go to Las Vegas, but felt she had no choice. She tried living in California for work and commuting to Nevada on weekends, but that took a toll on her, much so that I received a "second call" that Joy had taken some substance and never wanted to wake up. Unfortunately, I was living in Virginia at the time and couldn't get to the West Coast. So I called her husband. When they found her, she was still alive. Joy was put on an involuntary psychiatric hold and admitted to a local hospital. She promised to go through counseling, so they released her the next day. Joy ended up moving to Las Vegas full time. She developed a gambling addiction that consumed her. Over the course of the next few years she tried to take her life several more times. She tried to slit her wrists. She tried to overdose. She locked herself in the garage with her car engine turned on. But she never called me until after it was all over. Sometimes it was days or weeks later.

One Sunday after I had talked to Joy on the phone, I called her husband, because I didn't know what to do for her anymore. Little did I know that this day would be the last time I would talk with her. That evening her husband called to tell me Joy had gone outside and shot herself in the head while he was at the store. I have no idea what transpired after my call with her husband. I felt like life had been sucked right out of me; I collapsed on the floor.

John was the love of my life. My soul mate. My other half. He was kind and funny. He "got" me. He made me happy. We had known each other for many years before we fell in love. When it hit, it was magical. We started on a road where we laughed, cried, and faced many ups and downs. Things moved forward. When you know you want to be with someone forever, you work to make it happen. We bought a townhouse and got engaged. Life together was good. Our kids all got along well, and they seemed to warm up to us as individuals and as a couple. Holidays were all about family. It was a wonderful life. Or at least I thought it was.

In all honesty, John had never really gotten over his divorce. His ex-wife's affair cut into him like a knife. He felt betrayed. He felt angry. He felt revengeful. Over time it started to consume him. He was mad at everything. If something had to do with his ex-wife or his kids or money, his blood would boil. You could see it. The anger escalated, and it started to affect our relationship. It seemed like a darkness had transformed him into someone I really didn't know anymore. Angry. Vengeful. Hurtful. It was hard to leave someone I loved so much, but there was nothing more I could do. He went his way and I went mine.

I moved back to California a year later. We corresponded and even saw each other a couple of times. John told me that at one point he had gone through surgery to repair a herniated disc in his neck. It left him in chronic pain, and I heard he had to go on disability. This must have been hard for him. John had been in law enforcement and the federal government for many years. He was proud of his career.

I heard later that John had turned to prescription medication and alcohol to numb the pain. I guess over time the pain became too much to bear. On the day it happened, my sister called and said she was going to stop by because she had something to tell me. I had no idea what it was about. When she told me John had committed suicide, I am not sure it registered. He couldn't have committed suicide. As a former cop, he abhorred suicide. He couldn't understand why someone would do that. It was just not his personality. But then I remembered my friend Joy and the fact that people who commit suicide are "not themselves" when they make that decision. The pain must have consumed him to the point where he just wanted to make it go away. It broke my heart to know John had been hurting so much. His mom told me later that he had been saying for at least a few months, "If anything happens to me, you need to.…" This means he had been planning it, which made it even worse.

How can you plan to die when you have two children, one who is about to graduate from college in a couple of weeks? What about his mom? How could he leave her alone? She moved to Virginia to be closer to him. Yet leave them he did. He left them with no understanding and wanting answers. But answers never came. Nothing ever came. Well, that's wrong, something came: extreme sadness and heartache, and it hasn't gone away.

*

BONNIE FORSHEY
Bonnie's son Billy
died in 1993 at age 16

My son Billy never made it through his teens. Our world was turned upside down due to suicide. I still do not know if it was intentional or not. There are so many unanswered questions. Billy was a very kind and funny soul. He was always giving his belongings to others who were less fortunate than him. That is what I remember most, his generosity. Billy could light up a room with his smile and blue eyes. You could never have a bad day with him around. He was my practical joker. He was flesh of my flesh, blood of my blood, and was my heart and soul.

On October 30, 1993, I lost him. He was sixteen, forever sixteen. I lost my sanity, and my self-identity. The person that I am now is not the same person I used to be. I have to wear a mask to fake my emotions, to pretend that everything is okay, when it will never be okay again.

I had no idea that Billy had written a will and given it to his friend. Even her parents were aware, but no one told me. Billy had gotten in trouble for cutting his arms in school, but I was never told. When I did see marks, he told me that it happened in his agriculture class when he was carrying cages. Billy started sleeping a lot. He told me it was because he stayed up too late. I never knew that it was because he had taken antidepressants out of the trashcan, his stepfather's old Sinequan pills. They were toxic, yet Billy was taking them. He had gotten involved with people who would later give him Valium and marijuana...I never knew until it was too late. I was a nurse, I should have known, should have seen, but I didn't.

Approximately one week prior to the loss of my son, I began feeling very anxious. I had very bad premonitions, and my heart knew that something was about to happen, but I never would have believed it would be the loss of my child. I worked the 3 to 11 p.m. shift that week, and I remember frantically calling my house at night to check on my son. I went as far as to clock out just to come home and check on him. It was out of my hands, and as those dreaded events unfolded, I could not do a thing to stop them.

I was at home when Billy came out of his room and opened his mouth to show me all the pills. He immediately drank a glass of water and ran into his bedroom, locking the door behind him. I immediately called 911 and then called Billy's father. His father had left us when Billy was a toddler, and didn't want to be bothered. As I called Billy's dad, I heard a faint voice cry out on the extension phone, "Dad, you will never have to worry about me again, I am dying." *Click.* I kicked Billy's door down and held him while waiting for the ambulance. I kissed him and told him how much I loved him. My last memories are horrific: waiting for the ambulance, Billy going unconscious in my arms...it was all too late.

We got to the ER, and I thought Billy would be fine. We treated overdoses on a daily basis, and they all recovered and went home. It was usually the gunshot victims who didn't make it. But I was wrong! I remember the doctor taking us back to a quiet room. I thought he was going to tell me that Billy was fine...wrong again. My whole world came crashing down when the doctor told me they did all they could, but Billy coded three times and was gone. We were led into the room where my precious child lay on a gurney. He was still intubated, and there was charcoal all over his face. His clothing had been cut off, and it was handed to me. He was forever still. Never again would I hear his laughter, or see his smiling blue eyes light up. I would never again hear the words "I love you, Mom," or hear him call me "Shorty." He had towered above me, and thought it was so funny. I was forever changed. I miss the very essence of his soul. I miss my child, but I celebrate his life. He was a wonderful child, friend and brother. I am thankful for the sixteen sweet years we had; I wouldn't have missed them for the world.

*

LAURA HABEDANK
Laura's brother Brian
died in 2010 at age 35

My life was irreversibly changed on October 13, 2010, when I received the call from my mom confirming that my brother had been found dead in his home. He had taken his own life.

I learned of his lifelong struggle with depression only five months earlier when he confided in me that he had attempted suicide twice before. I spent the following months regularly reaching out to him, arranging for therapy appointments and panicking each time a phone call or text went unanswered, fearing the worst. I felt so helpless being so far away. He was living in my home state of Minnesota, and I had relocated to Texas less than a year earlier. I was desperately trying to save his life, and even went so far as to ask Brian to promise me that he wouldn't hurt himself. He told me that was a promise he could not keep.

Throughout the day on October 13, Brian was not responding to any emails, text messages or phone calls. After a number of family members pieced details together, we determined that no one had been in contact with Brian since a week earlier. We made the decision to send the police to his home for a wellness check, and they confirmed our worst fears. The medical examiner said he had likely been dead nearly a week before he was found. My life was completely turned upside down, and I've spent the last five years learning to live in this "new normal."

One of the ways I cope is by writing letters to Brian; it helps me process my feelings and feel as though I'm still able to connect with him in a way. Here is the first letter I wrote him a few months after his death.

Dear Brian,

I'll never forget the last time I saw you. It was July 5, 2010. You brought me back to the airport after my visit home for Mom's birthday. The entire ride was so heartbreaking; I could feel it– your profound sadness. I tried to get you to talk about it but you kept changing the subject... so I let it be. I just wanted to spend time with you. I didn't want the ride to end; the closer we got to the airport the more anxious I grew. I didn't want to say goodbye to you– something was happening that made my heart ache for you but I couldn't put my finger on it exactly. You got out to help me with my bags, I gave you a hug and said, "Come visit me soon, okay?? See ya later, dude." Once inside the airport doors I allowed myself to turn around in time to see you driving away; I started sobbing because in my heart I knew I'd never see you again... and I didn't.

That part still haunts me– that I was so connected with you that I could sense that but yet I didn't feel it the moment you died. It will take me a lifetime to get past that an entire week passed before you were found. I felt like I let you down; not only did you die alone but you continued to lie there alone for a week while I went about my life. "He's gone, honey." Those are the first words I heard from Mom confirming that what we had hoped hadn't happened, really had. The nightmare began. For weeks I would call your cellphone several times a day just to hear your voicemail message; I worry that I'll forget the sound of your voice. I was a mess the first time I called your number after it was finally disconnected; it was like you had died all over again and the last remaining connection I had to hearing your voice again was gone.

I keep running through our life together over and over in my head. We were so close in age that we shared everything together; we experienced all stages of life at the same time: childhood... high school... college... jobs... everything. And we even liked each other enough to choose to be roommates as adults! I loved that we were not just brother and sister, but we were friends. We included each other in our circles of friends and activities. I keep trying to remember those things: our Sundays watching the Simpsons, you "singing" me the X-Files theme song, pizza and football games, and even you trying, very patiently, to teach me how to drive a manual transmission! You had the most amazing, contagious laugh and a very gentle spirit and are going to be missed by so many people- more than you could have ever imagined. It may not make sense but it feels like you have taken that past with you... and it also feels as though you have also taken my future as I never imagined it without you.

I often wonder how long it'll be before those memories bring me more joy than pain- because right now it hurts to think of them. My heart is broken! I find myself detaching from the world, I'm suffering from frequent panic attacks when the pain is just so strong it takes my breath away. I have become jealous of others who have siblings who are still here- and I'm hurt when I see them angry with each other. I am not the same person anymore; I feel so isolated, so different from everyone else. I can laugh... but have no true joy right now. I suppose some happiness will come back someday... but for now there's only a hole in my heart where you used to be.

Please know that I am not angry at you now... nor do I think I ever will be. I have been to that place myself before and fought my way back out. I know it wasn't a compulsive choice you made but rather the culmination of years and years of battling a crippling depression and you held on as long as you could- for us. I miss you and think of you every waking moment.

Instead of saying goodbye to you, since I know I'll see you again, I'll just say what we always said to each other- "See ya later, dude."

Your loving sister,

Laura

*

VICKI HECKROTH
Vicki's son Matthew
died in 2000 at age 17

I knew my son was having a tough time with things but, he always told me he was fine. But the mask he always wore he has now passed on to me. Matthew had attention deficit disorder, ADD, and had a hard time concentrating. The summer between his sophomore and junior years of high school, he wrecked two cars. I refused to buy him another.

Matt turned seventeen in August of that year, and he used his birthday money along with what he had saved from his job to buy his own car. Our only stipulation was that he had to get his own insurance, and he swore he did.

Matt worked with me at a restaurant. He bought his car on October 31, 2000. Three days later, on November 3, he was late for work. Of course I was concerned because my kids were never late. When he did get there, someone had dropped him off. No car. He told me he had been in another accident, the car was totaled, and the lady he hit was taken to the hospital, claiming back injuries. He had given the cops his insurance card, but we were told it was invalid. Matt had not paid for his insurance after all.

Not only was I upset, but the lady whom Matt hit was threatening a lawsuit. The DOT wanted both my son's and my husband's driver's licenses turned in because the car was in both their names, and there was no insurance. That was a very long weekend, with everyone upset.

On Monday, November 6, Matt went to school and I went to work. After work I went to get his car out of impound, and then had a couple of drinks with a friend. When I arrived home, Matt was in his room. I called him out and again asked about the insurance. He swore he had paid it. I didn't know what or whom to believe. I went to take a shower, leaving Matt in the living room. And then I heard a loud bang. Thinking I had left the screen door open, I came out of the bathroom and walked into a nightmare.

The screen door was fine, but the gun cabinet was open and Matt was no longer in the living room. I immediately went to his room with a sick feeling in my stomach. I found my son lying on the floor with the gun on his chest and a black ring under his chin. He had shot himself. When I raised his head to try to help him, the damage was beyond repair. My life changed forever.

My family will never be the same. I still have nightmares of that night. The vision was at the forefront of my thoughts. I am in therapy, and have started a group called GLASS both online and off to try to help others who are going through this and to talk to local agencies and schools to try to stop suicide.

My daughters have also been to hell and back. We reflect on everything we ever did or said that might have caused Matt's depression. Why didn't we see it? How could this have happened? I didn't smile or laugh for years; in fact, I barely do even now. I have ten grandchildren. Only one ever met her uncle. She was only five months at the time of his death, but has memories and says things to us that she should not know. Her story is printed in the book, *Heaven Talks to Children*, by Christine Duminiak.

I still spend countless hours and many nights in tears, wondering what my son would be like today. He was just a kid, a junior in high school, when he passed. He should have been a thirty-two-year-old adult with children and a wife of his own by now. Not only was I robbed of him, but of his future as well. When I hear of another suicide or talk with a suicidal teen, the memories come back as if the floodgates opened. Many times I have gotten so depressed that I could easily go join him. There are times when I feel like I died with him, and they just forgot to bury me.

Every day that I can get through is one more day with my loved ones here, but also one day closer to the day when I will be reunited with my son. Life has gone on, as I knew it would. But it will never be the same. I am forever changed. I lost many friends over Matt's death. I am not the fun-loving person I once was.

I am now a grieving mother. My main goal is to help other mothers from having to go through this alone. The first support group I went to was The Compassionate Friends. A gentleman there put his hand on my knee and said, "But your son chose to die; mine did not." I could not get out of there fast enough.

There were no support groups for just suicide at that time. In 2000 you still did not talk about it. It was something shameful. I was told my son was weak, a coward. That is NOT at all true. My son fought a hard battle within himself. He fought hard all his life, battling ADD and depression, which is a disease. It is a disease that can and does kill. Matt may have lost the battle, but I give him credit for fighting as long as he did. Since his death, I too suffer from major clinical depression and I know how hard it is to fight sometimes. I wear the same mask my son did. Pretending to be okay when inside Matt was being torn apart. That is me today.

*

MARLISE MAGNA
Marlise's fiancé Blaine
died in 2010 at age 36

I met Blaine about three years before his death through a friend on Facebook. We clicked immediately, and enjoyed engaging in happy banter and debates. He was involved at the time and so was I, so it was always aboveboard and just a good conversation. After almost two years of being friends, circumstances changed and we decided to meet up. Our first encounter was literally all of two minutes but we *knew* we were meant to be. After that we spent a lot of time together, although it wasn't easy. We didn't live near each other, and his ex-girlfriend, who is the mother of his son, caused a lot of problems. She withheld their son to punish Blaine, and I firmly believe this may be a pertinent factor in his decision to take his life. I so wish I could meet up with his little "T-man," as Blaine called him, and tell him how awesome the father was. We never had the chance to have kids together.

We were set to get married on 11/11/2011, it was a number that Blaine simply loved and insisted on. He then wanted to move to Bali and live an idyllic island life. Towards the end he would say many times, "Baby girl, I'm gonna kill myself. It's gonna be epic," and "See you on the other side." Blaine was a Microsoft certified systems engineer and always loved expanding his fields of knowledge. Music was another passion, one we shared. He was a huge lover of Pearl Jam, and often quoted their lyrics. Together, we had released a few tracks of trance-type music on iTunes. He also had an amazing penchant for writing. He loved scuba diving and often wrote stories about dives and finding black pearls (which I was apparently, to him). He loved coffee and his favorite food was chicken lasagna. He was a body training expert!

I knew in the week leading up to Blaine's death that he wasn't one hundred percent himself, but I never dreamed things would escalate. On the day Blaine took his life, he left me a few Facebook messages saying, "I love you baby girl." He was very quiet but I ascribed it to his erratic sleeping patterns and assumed he had fallen asleep in the morning hours. About 2 p.m. I received a text message saying to please call regarding Blaine, but it came from his phone number. Fear set in. I called and a close family friend answered and told me what had happened. At first I said that if Blaine wanted to end things with me, to just say so, and not make sick jokes. But it was no joke. I frantically started calling morgues to find Blaine and, once I got the details, I drank myself into a fitful sleep.

The next morning, I made the long and arduously heart-wrenching trip to the state morgue where all suicides go to be autopsied. I met Blaine's mom there for the first and only time. It was surreal, his family thought Blaine had made me up in his mind.

I wasn't allowed to see his body alone but the head of the morgue took pity and said if I waited until closing time, he would allow me a few minutes alone with Blaine. Imagine seeing the man you love, your best friend and lover, lying cold and lifeless, still blood splattered from the autopsy. I died a million times over and then some.

From that day forward, it was surviving day to day until the funeral. Blaine's family told people he had suffered a heart attack. My life stopped after that. I became totally depressed and tried taking my own life. I ended up under psychiatric supervision for three weeks. For months after, I partied hard, I guess to numb the pain. I became a total insomniac and suffered great anxiety and depression. Blaine was an only child and I cannot imagine his mom's agony. She has been left utterly alone.

My life has never been the same. Yet, I thank Blaine for sharing his time on earth with me. I thank him for enriching my life and broadening my horizons and encouraging me to be the authentic me, and loving me without condition. I thank him for being there for the good and the bad. I thank him for changing my life path.

I thank God for lending him to us for a little bit. We always said "two hearts beating as one," and "two against the world baby, two against the world."

To quote "Just Breathe," one of his favorite Pearl Jam songs: "Nothing you would take. Everything you gave. I hope until I die... Meet you on the other side."

From Blaine to me:

Love at first sight is a fantasy.
The make believe or the imaginary.
To some it's a gift that becomes real.
When the imaginary dream becomes real,
the ecstatic joy and freedom is a rare gem,
that few get to share.
I'm glad that I know,
that I have found that gem.
In you.
You are my fantasy and God willing my reality.
I Love you, mind, body and soul.
Under the sun, the moon, the stars.

DJ Zer0.1 and Mia Magna, forever. See you on the other side.

*

MARCELLA MALONE
Marcella's brother Michael
died in 2014 at age 20

Just fifteen months younger than me, it was inevitable that Michael and I would grow up really close to each other. Up until middle school we were best friends. Many of our friends were even the same. I was into his favorite activities, like participating in a variety of sports, hunting, fishing, and select video games (they were never my strong suit). He traded off and did crafts and played house with me. We had outside friends, but at the end of the day all we needed was each other.

When Michael was in middle school and I in high school, we began to spend less time around each other, but remained close. Until the end, we took on caregiving roles with each other. I spoiled him by cooking, driving him around, helping with chores, picking up his tab, packing for him. In turn, he protected me, making sure I was always happy and safe. We told each other most things.

Following high school and the events that led up to Michael not being able to follow his dream of playing college football, he went through a brief down period, but he had seemed to be doing much better the past year or so. He was back to his goofy, fun-loving, super caring self who strove to live life to its fullest.

Michael was working with our dad in Operating Engineers Union Local 324 and making great money for his age. In late March we had returned from a week-long family vacation in Florida. We had a great time and I was thankful for the time I was able to spend with him, as life made these occurrences much less frequent than I had liked. Everything seemed to be going well for Michael; he seemed happy.

Fast-forward a couple of weeks to Monday, April 14, 2014. It started out as a normal day. I texted Michael in the morning to make plans to go with him to pick out my baby shower present and talk about the rebuilding of the local FFA barn. Michael was helping my dad paint the upstairs of the house.

When I got out of class, I checked my Facebook page and noticed an unusual post from Michael: "To all those who love me, thank you for showing me what love is." I immediately knew something was wrong. I called and texted Michael repeatedly with no reply. I then began trying to reach his friends and our family to see if anyone knew anything. Everyone was just as worried, and many were out searching for Michael. I was two hours away and had class in the morning. I felt completely helpless. I tried to talk to those close to me about my fears, as it was unlike Michael to behave like that, but everyone seemed to feel I was overthinking it.

I tried to stay positive and to remember a couple of years earlier when Michael was down and would just go hide out at the lake or a friend's house to take a break. I hoped that was true again this time. I went to take a bath to relax, but when I got out I didn't even have time to dry off before I heard the phone ring. It was our dad. Hoping for good news, I quickly answered the phone. The pain in his voice was unbearable as he said, "Michael's dead. He shot himself." The police had found his body and had just come to notify my parents. I immediately dropped my phone and towel; I couldn't believe what I had heard. I was speechless and couldn't even produce a tear. My roommate heard the phone fall and came to check on me. She helped me pack what I needed, as my brain was too scattered for even such a simple task.

During the last snowfall of the year I drove to my parents' house. Through the tears, I sat with them, my older brother and my sister-in-law in complete silence as we prepared for the hardest week of our lives. None of our lives would ever be the same.

My brain was overwhelmed with questions of "why" and "what if" for a long time. It's hard to explain how it has changed my life. It's almost a year and a half later, and I still struggle daily. My anxiety is definitely much greater, as well as my struggle to trust others, as I feel like they will never understand my emotions. However, it has also given me a passion toward a future career path, and made me much more perceptive to the emotions of others.

No matter the pain I feel, each day I make it a point to try to make others smile, because you never know what others are going through. Through all the bad I found good, because I know Michael wouldn't want to see me in pain. The hardest thing is remembering that I will never see him. His nephew, whom Michael was so excited about, will never get the chance to meet him. But life must go on, and for Michael, my guardian angel, I have to do my best to "live big."

*

JULIE MJELVE
Julie's husband Cameron
died in 2011 at age 42

In 2009 my husband returned to university. In 2010, his second year, he seemed to have more difficulty maintaining the work and scheduling of his courses. Over the Christmas break he seemed different, a bit off from his usual self. Perhaps a little depressed, but nothing that raised any immediate concern. I chalked this up to the stresses of university.

On January 31, 2011, our youngest daughter was born with a diagnosis of Down syndrome. Adding one more stressor to Cameron's life turned out to be more than he was able to cope with.

On the evening of July 21, the police rang my doorbell. They informed me that my husband had committed suicide by shooting himself in the heart. I was in shock at first, and didn't believe they had the right person. They said they found a black truck parked in his parents' driveway. We didn't own a black truck and Cameron's parents were out of town, so I thought it couldn't have been him. But they insisted they did have the right person, even if the vehicle description was wrong.

As I pressed for more details, I learned that Cameron was found in his parents' front yard by a construction worker building a house nearby. The worker heard the gunshot and, having experienced suicide in his own family, knew what was going on. He ran to my husband's side and called 911. Although my husband was still alive in the ambulance, he did not survive. I found it very comforting to know that he did not die alone, even though it was in the presence of strangers, and I'm so thankful for those who came to his aid.

Cameron's suicide has changed my life dramatically. There are physical challenges, such as raising children by myself, and emotional challenges, such as dealing with the sometimes thoughtless comments of others. However, all these challenges have served to make me a stronger and, hopefully, more thoughtful and attentive person.

I have learned much about the grieving process, and how important it is. I found that others would forget very quickly that not only was I grieving, but I was also dealing with the traumatic nature of his death, as well as trying to figure out how to help three very small children understand death and grieve in a way appropriate for their age. Because of this, I found it necessary for myself to really engage in the mourning part of the grieving process, something we don't do very well in North America, and yet it is so very important.

Going through this experience has also changed my life, in that I now have the opportunity to comfort others who have experienced loss as well. A good friend whose husband passed away unexpectedly with a heart condition called me right away, knowing I was the only person who would understand what she was going through. It was difficult. I relived it with her. The emotions, the challenges of knowing what to say as she struggled to tell her daughter that her daddy had died. But I was so glad to be able to be there for her, to just be beside her and do nothing but cry with her, as someone who knows the pain.

I have also had to struggle to deal with the stigma associated with suicide. Although I feel as though I personally understand the mental health issues that lead a person toward suicide, I find that there are still many who do not, and still place quite a lot of judgments on suicide.

Even four years later I'm only just now becoming able to tell others that my husband died due to suicide. Before, I just couldn't bring myself to say it, it was like living it all over again. Knowing how and what to tell the children has also been very difficult. They were very young when their dad passed away. I chose to tell them that he died because he got sick, with the intention of telling them when they're older that the type of sickness he died from is mental health disease. And, I have done just that now. They know it was suicide, and we have talked about what suicide means. They know that it's a bad choice, made because the brain is sick and not thinking correctly. Most important, we have talked about what to do when we are feeling sad and depressed, that the depression makes it difficult for us to make the right choices and so we must seek out help.

Although it has been a very difficult experience to go through, having to face these situations and judgments head-on has helped form my thoughts about it in a more concise way. I hope to be able to use this personal experience in a way that can educate others to the real issues going on for those who commit suicide. It's more than just an act when someone commits it; it is a sickness, and a very serious sickness which requires medical attention. So although it has been a difficult time, I feel that I have grown as a person, and have come out stronger as a result.

*

BRIDGET PARK
Bridget's brother Austin
died in 2008 at age 14

My brother was never the stereotypical suicidal person who wore black or slit his wrists, but rather was very good at being just the opposite. He was his freshman class president and a football player whom all the girls drooled over. I was his dorky younger sister who wore matching sweat outfits, had greasy hair, and embarrassed her older brother at any given moment.

It was a cold November day on the ranch, and just like every Saturday, my brother and I were assigned chores by my parents. I could tell that Austin was high-strung that day or a little less patient, but it was nothing I thought too much about. After a long day of work, we were covered in cow manure and dirt. Since it was Saturday, there was a chance to go to church that evening and to attend the 4:30 p.m. mass that was offered in our small hometown. Being the devout Catholic family that we were, we never missed church. So when we finished chores, we all rushed inside to clean up. However, I guess we didn't hurry fast enough, because when it was time for us to leave, Austin was still in the shower and I had yet to go. My parents, for the first time, let my brother and me miss church. But of course they left us with a list of chores they wanted to be completed by their return.

After my shower, Austin and I set out to start our first chore of the evening, which was to clean the kitchen. There was not much to do other than a few dishes and to wipe the counters. I was not really in a hurry, but Austin sure was. I had never seen him clean so fast before with such determination. Girls and friends kept texting and calling him, asking if he wanted to go out that evening. He just ignored the buzzes of his phone and continued to wipe the counter furiously. At this point I just assumed he was having an off day. As we finished the chore Austin kept saying, "I want to watch TV in Mom and Dad's room," repeatedly. I thought nothing of this other than that he wanted the big TV and the big comfy bed. I followed him to the door of my parents' bedroom and said, "Let me know if you need anything, Austin." I failed to hear the lock of the door click behind him. About fifteen minutes later, I received a call from our cousin asking to speak with Austin. I left my room, passed our living room, turned down the TV I had blasted with my favorite show, and started toward my parent's bedroom. I reached for the doorknob and started to turn it, but it was locked. I casually thought that Austin was just on the phone with a girl or was dancing to his latest favorite tune. I opened a door that led outside and was across from a second door into the bedroom. I immediately saw something red through the glass door. I approached the second bedroom door and there I saw my older brother on his back and a rifle next to him. I had never seen someone look so pale before, so translucent. I fell to the ground in fear, thinking that someone was there at my home, because my brother would never harm himself in any manner, so it had to be someone else's doing. I never imagined that something so terrible, so tragic, would ever happen to my picture-perfect family.

For years it was a foggy memory until I allowed it to be translucent. Once I did so, I was able to begin healing and growing. I was able to not be ashamed of my brother and my past, because I learned that by helping and sharing my story with others, it just happens to be the way I grieve best and most healthily.

*

GRACE YOUNG

Grace's son Jack died

in 2007 on his 27th birthday

I've always thought that motherhood was something I did well, enjoyed, something God had planned for me. I loved my children, and encouraged them to share their thoughts and feelings. I was raised by a nurse mom, so I was educated about parenting, good health, nutrition, and keeping faith a part of family life.

Our children were smart, handsome, intelligent, and caring souls. It was hard when they moved out of the nest, first Jack after he graduated from high school in 1999. He moved to Kansas with a few friends to pursue his music and his art. We had always encouraged his love of music, and his many bands in high school rattling our windows as they practiced in our basement.

We encouraged our children not to drink alcohol, as our family has a history of alcoholism. Since we were not drinkers, it was not something they favored, thankfully. But Jack's foray into the world of rock 'n' roll often found him nursing a beer or something harder, much to my chagrin.

Jack left Kansas after a bit, and moved to New York City. His brother Ben was attending film school there, so they shared an apartment. It was then that Ben noticed that Jack was drinking more than normal, seemed to keep some shady friends, and dabbled in drug use. Ben tried to talk some sense into Jack, and told us of Jack's difficulties keeping up with his bills. Ben noticed that Jack would often drink heavily, produce some scary art pieces, and seemed depressed when yet another girlfriend broke up with him. Jack was a very handsome young man, and had many girlfriends, often from overseas as internet chatting became more prevalent.

Jack left to live with a sweet girl in England for a year or so, then returned, heartbroken again. A few times Ben called us to complain that Jack wasn't pitching in with the housework and finances, and was concerned that Jack's depression was worsening. During their time on their own, we spoke to the boys nearly every other day, giving them suggestions about problems, checking up on their lives, and trying to stay in the loop as they grew into responsible young men.

When Ben graduated from film school, they left New York City and moved to Putnam, Connecticut, as their grandmother had given them her four-family apartment building. This was a great situation for everyone, as Mom could live in one of the apartments, Ben and Jack could share the largest apartment, and they would have the income from the other two apartments. They both continued to work, and Jack continued his musical career, working part time and playing music at night. Once again, though, Ben and Jack clashed on many points similar to the problems in New York City, and it was decided that Jack would move to Pittsburgh, Pennsylvania, with his Swiss fiancée to work with a friend on his art business. They would work on their art and still pursue their music scene. We all helped to pack up Jack's van and helped him with the move to Pennsylvania. Jack seemed to be doing well. He and his fiancée seemed very happy, and although he was still drinking somewhat, life seemed to be moving along more smoothly now that Jack was with his fiancée and no longer living with Ben.

In the middle of one night in February 2006, Jack's friend called to tell me that Jack seemed to be out of control with his drinking, and he was worried. I immediately flew to Pittsburgh to find out what was really going on. Jack and his fiancée were struggling, both were drinking heavily, and Jack's depression was very apparent. We decided to drive back to Putnam to see if we could get him into a treatment program.

My mother was going to be celebrating her seventy-fifth birthday with our whole family, so it was great to have them both here for her big party. Everyone on my side of the family was able to see him, and we all spoke candidly about Jack's struggles, and brainstormed together about how to get him the help he needed. We talked, we cried, we screamed and prayed, and earnestly started looking for suitable treatment for him. Sadly, because of a lack of beds locally, and due to Jack's lack of insurance, we were turned down by several local mental health facilities. In the end, Jack and his fiancée had to get back to Pittsburgh. They said they would go through their city's social services department to get him into a program in Pennsylvania. We kept in close contact, hoping they would find a facility who could help Jack, and we encouraged them to attend AA and find a church. The day before Jack's twenty-seventh birthday, I called to wish him a happy birthday, and he told me that his fiancée had gone to Switzerland to renew her green card. He seemed happy, and we talked and laughed for a while. I never would have believed what would happen the very next day. I was studying for my sign language final at our local college, having learned an E.E. Cummings poem, "I Carry Your Heart," for my final exam. When I went home from work for lunch, the phone rang. It was Jack's friend in Pittsburgh. He said, "Jack is gone." I said, "What do you mean, Jack's gone?" He said, "He hanged himself. I can't talk, the police are here, they will call you soon."

The howl that was released from my gut still rings in my ears. Sure enough, the next call was from the police. Jack was dead by hanging on his twenty-seventh birthday. I wasn't able to reach my husband at his work, and frantically drove back to my job, hysterical. My boss was able to contact my husband and my son Ben. The medical examiner called next, and he was so kind. "I have your son, I have secured his apartment, and I will make sure he makes it home safely."

We buried Jack the day before Mother's Day, and I remember sitting and opening the hundreds of sympathy cards on that day. We left the next day to drive out to empty Jack's apartment and bring his things home. It was eerie, walking into his basement apartment, wondering how he could have hanged himself in such a small place. We found the cord of his vacuum cut, and a small chair under the light fixture in the hallway. Our lives were forever changed.

A few weeks later, Jack's friends came to us and said they wanted to have a music benefit in his honor, to bring families together to learn the signs of depression and suicide. And from this, Particle Accelerator, named after a song Jack penned, was born. In the last nine years we have raised over forty thousand dollars for United Services, our local mental health organization. It is a fitting legacy for our beautiful son, the mixture of music and love to save lives. May God bless all the suicide angels.

CHAPTER TWO

THE AFTERMATH

*Somehow, even in the worst of times, the tiniest
fragments of good survive. It was the grip in which
one held those fragments that counted.
-MELINA MARCHETTA*

Following loss by suicide, the first questions we often ask ourselves
are: How am I going to survive this? How can I function when I
have no feeling or when those sensations are so strong they
threaten to paralyze me? How can I cope? There we stand in the
aftermath, feeling vulnerable and often ravaged with fear. How do
we survive?

*

KAYLA ARNOLD
Kayla's uncle Tim
died in 2001 at age 34

During the initial aftermath of finding out that my uncle killed
himself, I cried a lot. I was shocked and really had no clue as to how
to process what I had just been told. I was a twelve-year-old who
didn't even know what suicide was, let alone how to wrap my head
around how a man I loved so much could choose to leave me and
the rest of his family willingly.

33

I had no clue as to how to start to heal. I didn't want to be bothered or be around anyone. All I wanted to do was sit around and cry! I found myself very angry, I got so mad when everyone would come up to me and apologize and say, "I'm sorry for your loss." I was dealing with trying to comprehend something that made no sense to me, and people saying that angered me.

I remember that my uncle died on a Thursday. The Saturday after he died we had a baby shower for my aunt. The one thing I remember was getting very mad and running off down the hallway. I was so mad that everyone kept telling me they were sorry! I didn't want to hear it, I didn't want them to keep telling me that; they didn't know what I was going through. They didn't understand that one of my favorite people had been taken from me, and they had no clue about the pain I was feeling.

The aftermath was horrible, draining and exhausting. It took years to be able to talk about Uncle Tim without crying and breaking down. I sometimes feel like I am still dealing with the aftermath fourteen years later, and it still doesn't seem real.

*

EMILY BARNHARDT
Emily's friend and roommate Hannah
died in 2014 at age 20

The level of devastation and confusion after a loss like this is completely beyond description. There are no adequate words to describe the deep ocean of ache that washes over you as relentlessly as waves are washed over the shore. Looking back, I only remember a series of blackened days. Moving through each day felt like moving through concrete. I couldn't understand why everyone's world was still turning while mine had come to a shuddering halt. I wasn't there; I was suspended in a world that wasn't reality, a world where Hannah was still alive and I couldn't understand why everything was unfolding as if she had died.

I slipped in and out of denial, wondering why I hadn't talked to her or seen her and thinking she must be on vacation. Our minds go into survival mode after a devastating trauma. Our mind protects us in a way, because it knows we can't possibly bear the full extent of the pain all at once. So our mind gives us doses of reality a little at a time. Even so, those little doses of reality left me feeling as if I were stumbling across a seemingly never-ending field of landmines. I never knew when that next dose would erupt.

I often sat alone and scared in our apartment night after night, feeling Hannah's presence all around me. The silence was deafening. I woke up each morning, and for a second everything felt normal. For a second, I'd forgotten. Then it would hit me and I would remember. Those moments of forgetting and remembering again were brutal. I'd pull the covers up over my head and curl up underneath them, as if I could hide and shield myself from reality.

The never-ending and unanswered questions plagued me day in and day out. I dreaded sleeping, because every time I closed my eyes, it began, that tape reel in my mind, playing over and over the events of that night, my role in it, the unanswered questions, the haunting images of her dying the way she did, and the memories.

I saw Hannah everywhere I went. Every moment and activity of my day felt saturated with memories of her. Her death over-shadowed everything. I volleyed between wanting to be around people and wanting to be alone. I felt overwhelmed and suffocated being around people, yet crippled by a pervasive, aching loneliness when I was by myself. Somehow it felt like Hannah's pain was transferred to me, like catching a virus. In my strive to find answers and understand why, it was as if I had picked up the heavy burden she was carrying. The anguish and despair she carried that night became my own in a way, and it terrified me. I couldn't escape it; the constant exposure to the subject of suicide and the weight it carries weighed heavily on me. I look back and don't know how I made it through the initial aftermath of her death.

Life and its responsibilities and obligations swirled around me, and I simply did the best I could to withstand the pace. I know the only reason I survived those initial months is because I clung to my faith in Jesus for dear life; He was and is my only unfailing source of strength and hope. I berated myself for things I wasn't doing and ways I should be "grieving better." But I learned how essential it is to celebrate my victories. As in most cases of grief, there were some people in my life who said critical things about how I was grieving, but they weren't in my shoes. They didn't know how much strength it took to get out of bed some days or just to go to the grocery store, let alone a social event. It was crucial for me to learn how to validate myself and be proud of myself for the victories I had, regardless of others' opinions. I had to learn to be empathetic toward myself and ride each wave as it came.

We, as humans, are such analytical beings. We always want to know *how* and *how long*. I found peace in continually reminding myself *as long as it takes*. I gave myself compassion and cut myself some slack in areas where I wasn't performing well. I didn't rebuke myself if I stayed in bed for two days. I tried to find a balance in allowing myself the permission to grieve in the way my body and mind needed to, while also being aware and cautious of where to draw the line before it became unhealthy. I did the best I could, and sometimes that's all we can ever really do. And doing the best you can with what you have, in an unbearably difficult situation like this, is something to be proud of.

*

CHRISTINE BASTONE
Christine's sister Elizabeth
died in 2012 at age 38

That first night I went online, and searched for how to deal with this tragedy. I also joined two Yahoo groups. I was very, very busy for about the next two weeks. I wasn't deliberately busy; that's usually just the nature of death, I think. But I believe it did help.

There was discussion about whether we would go to the memorial service. There was packing, and making all the arrangements to be out of town for a few days. There was the long two-day drive up to Ohio from Florida, and then there was getting situated in our motel room once we got there. There was seeing my sister's body, saying what I wanted to say to her, and watching my mother's anguish over the loss of her youngest child...her baby.

There was helping to write Liz's online obituary for the funeral home's website. There was going to the florist, and helping to pick out flowers for my sister. There was going to the cemetery where she would be buried. There was helping to pick out her tombstone.

Since we ended up being there a few more days than we expected, I even got to do a few things I had been wanting to do for a while, such as going to a lake that I used to live right across from. There was meeting old friends at church. There was writing my first, and so far only, eulogy. There was getting ready for the memorial service. There was the memorial service, and the get-together afterward. There was visiting with my dad's sister, and catching up with her. And before I knew it, there was the very long drive home.

Like I said, I was busy! But I was okay. My appetite was a little off, and I couldn't sleep for more than four hours a night, but otherwise I think I handled it well. As is normal in such situations, we had a lot of support during those first few weeks. And of course I was also still in shock. So it wasn't until I got back home again and it felt like everyone had disappeared that things got a lot tougher to handle, and when my grief really began.

*

SHARON EHLERS
Sharon's best friend Joy died in 2009 at age 52
Sharon's former fiancé John died in 2012 at age 59

When I heard that Joy had killed herself, I collapsed on the floor. I was numb. It was a Sunday night, and there was no way I could sleep. Every time I closed my eyes I would see her. See her taking a gun and putting it to her head. Why Joy? Why? I left for Las Vegas a few days later. I needed to see her one more time. I needed to be with her "stuff." Maybe it would smell like her so it seemed like she was there.

When I got there it was tough. I saw the note in lipstick on the bathroom mirror: "Thank you, friends and family, for being there for me." Okay, that was sarcastic, not heartfelt. So she thought we hadn't been there for her. And since "friends" came before "family," maybe it was one "friend" in particular. Me. Our conversation had been fine when we spoke on Sunday. What happened or what was said afterward to make her kill herself? Still in the bathroom, I noticed the bullet hole in the window. I traced it with my eyes to the wall on the other side where it had lodged. I walked outside. The hole in the window was low, so that meant she had been sitting on the ground outside the window when it happened. I sat in the spot where I thought she had sat, and I cried.

I then walked back into the house and went straight for Joy's closet. I walked in and it still smelled like her perfume. I soaked it in. It was so comforting to smell her. I cried some more. Eventually I asked her husband if I could go to the funeral home to see her. He said no. He thought I wouldn't be able to deal with how she looked. I didn't care. I needed to see her one last time. I begged, but he was adamant. So I found my own way to mourn. I went to Joy's favorite store, Wal-Mart, and walked up and down the aisles. I did that for a long time. She loved that store. We could spend hours there just going up and down the aisles. We were great shoppers. Being in her "space" was very cathartic for me. It brought me comfort.

Once my sister told me about John's death, I was numb. Since I was in California and he died in Virginia, I tried to see what I could find on the internet. I finally found an emergency responder site that showed that a Medevac helicopter had been sent to our old address. That meant he had still been alive when they found him. My heart stopped. I reached out to friends back in Virginia to see what they knew. Eventually the local police called me, because we still owned the townhouse together. The officer was very respectful and answered all my questions. As he spoke it was like I was in a dream. I could picture the basement. I could picture the chair. A chair that I had bought John. I could picture him lying on the floor. I could see the notes they said he had left all over the house. It was a bad dream playing over and over. It felt like I was there when it happened. I thanked the officer and hung up. The hardest part was telling my children. John had been in our lives for a while. They grew up with him. They loved him. With Joy having committed suicide two years earlier, it was terrifying to think that I now had to tell them that John had too. Two people they knew and loved. The first thing my youngest daughter said was, "How did he die?" It was like she knew. I told her it was suicide. I told her that John shot himself. She was devastated. They were all devastated. I was beyond devastated. All we could do was cry.

The days that followed were like being in a fog. I don't really remember what was happening other than feeling disconnected from life. I spoke with John's mom and she gave me more information about what had been going on with him in the preceding months. She asked me so many questions that I couldn't answer. She asked me about John's bank accounts and safe deposit box. She asked me if he had a will. She asked me about the townhouse and the mortgage. John had left no information on anything. It was all too much. If he had planned it, why didn't he leave everything in order? What impacts was his suicide going to have on those of us left behind? It was hard enough trying to deal with the pain of his death.

*

BONNIE FORSHEY
Bonnie's son Billy
died in 1993 at age 16

I was horrified. I can remember the details of that day perfectly. I cried all the time, and shut the door to his room. I just couldn't believe that this was real. It felt like a nightmare.

I lived at the cemetery. I would go out there and lie on top of Billy's grave and cry. Then I would go home, and go into his room and cry. Billy was such a giving and kind young man, and I knew that he would want his belongings to go to his friends. Billy's best friend was very poor, and his mother didn't work. So I called him to come over and I gave him all of Billy's clothing, shoes, jewelry, etc. I knew Billy would have wanted me to do that, and it made me feel good.

*

LAURA HABEDANK
Laura's brother Brian
died in 2010 at age 35

It doesn't feel appropriate to say I was in "shock" because to be honest, I wasn't all that surprised that my brother ended his own life. But I just felt completely numb. I spent the next few months in a complete fog. I couldn't sleep through the night, I didn't feel like eating, I was experiencing racing thoughts of guilt and panic, and I felt physically ill most of the time. My own existing depression was shoved into high gear, and I responded by drinking too much, not answering my phone for anyone but my mom, and I recall endless hours lying on my right side, on my bed, and staring up at the silhouette of the trees outside my window against the bright blue sky and being so confused as to how it could look so beautiful out there and how the world seemed to keep moving on without me when I felt so exceedingly empty inside.

I spent so much time going over each and every detail of our last conversations and interactions, as if searching for a way to go back and get a "do-over," and possibly reach a different outcome. I was tormenting myself over all of the "what ifs" and the "if onlys" that my mind was a constant windstorm of self-doubt and self-blame for my brother's decision. I was obsessed with finding answers that in fact would never be found. I tried desperately to gain access to his cellphone, email and other account passwords, thinking if only I could just see the last email he ever sent or the last text he ever sent or received, or find out how he was able to obtain the illegal substances he ingested that resulted in his death then perhaps I'd be able to get some of the answers that I so desperately needed. I knew that the answers to those questions wouldn't bring my brother back, but I foolishly thought that they might bring me some comfort. In the end, all the frustratingly fruitless searching only left a bigger hole in my heart. I became obsessed with researching details that could only serve to bring more pain to myself, such as endlessly combing the internet for pictures and details about decomposition and the substances that would later be revealed to have been found in Brian's system. I wanted to know what he looked like when they found him. I needed to know who out there contributed to his death by either selling him those controlled substances or by posting the instructions online that describe the correct amounts to use, the correct combination to use, and in what order to ingest them. It took me a very long time to realize that, in the end, no one else was responsible for it. If it hadn't been this way, Brian would have found another way to do it. I just hoped that he didn't experience a great deal of physical pain.

I withdrew from the world. I did what I had to do to get by, such as getting myself to work and all, but I felt absolutely nothing; no connection to anyone. It felt pointless, really. No one could possibly understand the magnitude of the agony I was experiencing, so why bother? I had absolutely no patience for the seemingly trivial things going on with those around me. Hearing a coworker complain how "life sucked so much" because his or her car was in the shop was just more than I could handle. I was always on the verge of telling everyone around me, "My brother just killed himself!!! I'll tell you how much life sucks." Friends expressed their desire to have the "old Laura" back. That really hurt. I knew the "old me" wasn't ever coming back; you can't experience a loss of that magnitude and not be irreversibly changed. I wanted to know that I would still be loved, accepted and supported even in the new, broken form I was taking because I knew that from then on I would never, ever be the same.

*

VICKI HECKROTH
Vicki's son Matthew
died in 2000 at age 17

I got through the initial aftermath with the support of family and friends. My doctor put me on anxiety medication and antidepressants right away. I couldn't sleep or eat without them. All I wanted to do was sit in Matt's room and cry. There were sounds coming from my body that were not even human. They were more like animal howls. I hated everyone and everything. I blamed myself, yet I also blamed everyone else. I went on autopilot. I did the things I needed to do just so I wouldn't crash again.

I felt like I had died too and they just forgot to bury me.

Planning your own child's funeral is just not right. They are supposed to bury us; it's not supposed to be this way. My whole world went topsy-turvy. I drank a lot. The beer plus my medication dulled my feelings. The pain was not so great, because I couldn't feel it. Then when I did sober up, it felt like a body slam. I had to grieve all over again, and this time without everyone around to console me.

*

MARLISE MAGNA
Marlise's fiancé Blaine
died in 2010 at age 36

Honestly, I couldn't face the initial aftermath. I resorted to handfuls of pills, copious amounts of alcohol, and eventually a suicide attempt, which landed me in intensive care in a hospital. After I was classified with what would be called a nervous breakdown, I went for a three-week-long psychotherapy clinic, which helped a lot. During my stay his aunt let me know he was being cremated at that time. I never did speak to anyone in his family after that.

*

MARCELLA MALONE
Marcella's brother Michael
died in 2014 at age 20

The initial aftermath was a giant mix of shock, pain, and questions. I stayed with my parents from the night it happened until the day following the funeral. A week full of planning, chaos, meeting with detectives because of the gunshot, accusations, and lots of love. That last part got me through it. The love I had for my unborn child helped me take care of myself and stay calm, because he deserved that. The love of the countless family and friends who traveled to spend the days with us and make sure we didn't have to worry about things like food and cleaning made it easier to get by each moment.

The most important lives were those of my parents and my older brother and his fiancée who were also expecting their first child. We had to work together and take care of one another as we learned how to accept the shocking reality that Michael was really gone. The simplicity of having someone to sit with me so I wasn't alone in my grief was the most powerful. Nothing anyone said could have helped. Their just being there like a rock was the best. It is a time when you really find out who is there for you. As the week progressed, it also helped to share stories about the amazing young man Michael was with family and friends. Memories were all we had left so we had to cherish them.

When I returned home, it was more difficult to remember to take care of myself. I focused on the arrival of my child in July to keep my mind off the heartache. When I did break down, I was lucky to have an amazing roommate to comfort me through my nightmares, as well as my boyfriend to talk to me when I needed it. I also found it very helpful to remain close with Michael's good friends, as it helped keep his spirit alive for me. At the end of each day I'm still learning to cope. It's an evolving process.

*

JULIE MJELVE
Julie's husband Cameron
died in 2011 at age 42

The initial aftermath was very difficult. One of the things I did was refrain from telling the children right away. I took a day to find out what was the best way to tell them. It sounds strange to talk about this in a section about surviving the aftermath, but it was an important piece that made the rest of the aftermath a little more bearable.

Because I had taken that time to think things through, I didn't say anything I had to go back on, but instead I said things that I could build upon. A lot of my survival has centered around my children, because they were so small when my husband passed away. At the time they were three years old, two years old, and five months old. So a lot of my survival in the initial aftermath was simply that: survival. There wasn't much more that I could do other than take care of the children.

Surviving meant we made it out of the house to a playground, even if it took us all day to get there. Surviving meant we made it to school or to church, not that we were on time or prepared, just that we made it. Surviving meant I got supper made. I survived by not even trying to get my kids to sit at a table. We all sat in front of the TV with kid-sized lawn chairs and little trays for their plates. Not my ideal way to share supper with a family, but I had to survive.

Surviving the fact that my husband committed suicide has not been easy either. I felt I had to talk about all the events that led up to his death over and over and over again. I needed to analyze every decision I had made leading up to the events that Cameron found too stressful to cope with anymore. I went for counseling, and went often in the initial phases. I really needed someone to talk with who wouldn't get tired of hearing me question everything again and again.

I also coped by making what I called a "truth journal." For every action on my part where I questioned if I had done the right thing, I countered it with "the truth" about the situation and the choices that my husband made. Although people talk about the aftermath being the first few weeks and months, for me I found that the aftermath lasted years. It's only now, four and a half years later, that I feel like the "aftermath" is over and that I am coming out of the initial crisis of it. I think part of the coping has come from simply recognizing that it does take a lot longer than society traditionally gives us.

*

GRACE YOUNG
Grace's son Jack
died in 2007 on his 27th birthday

The pain in my heart was excruciating after my son's suicide on his birthday. Telling my mother and my husband's mother was heartbreaking. As they heard about it, family came around to comfort us, but the tears were constant. The same refrain, "Jack hanged himself on his birthday," was all my numb brain could process. I remember thinking that Jack could hear my thoughts, and was part of my heart again, where he was created.

Jack's wake and funeral brought more than 400 people. We had to travel to Pennsylvania to empty his apartment and pick up his car. I was saddened that the people in his building wouldn't even speak to us. Even when we asked them if they knew Jack, they just walked away without a word.

There was a huge storm on our way back, and our town was littered with limbs and leaves, torn apart, just like our hearts. The power was out, and we lit candles to carry Jack's things back into his old room. It seemed a fitting tribute.

*

CHAPTER THREE

THE FUNERAL

Some are bound to die young. By dying young a person stays young in people's memory. If he burns brightly before he dies, his brightness shines for all time. -UNKNOWN

For many the funeral represents the end while for others it marks the beginning of something eternal. Regardless of whether we mourn the absence of our child's physical body or celebrate the spirit that continues on, planning the funeral or memorial service in the aftermath of suicide presents emotionally-laden challenges shared by many.

*

KAYLA ARNOLD
Kayla's uncle Tim
died in 2001 at age 34

My grandparents, my mom and dad, and one of my other uncles planned Uncle Tim's funeral. Since I was so young, I didn't play much of a part in the planning of the funeral, but I do remember the visitation. At the visitation we sat with the pastor and we all shared memories of Uncle Tim, and the pastor used our memories in the service.

I also remember that when we got there and went up to see my uncle, they had his bandana on wrong, so my dad fixed it. My uncle always had the top button of his jeans undone, and the funeral workers had buttoned it, so my dad also undid that. Uncle Tim was wearing a University of Michigan shirt, his blue jeans and his bandana. We made sure Uncle Tim would be laid to rest just like he loved to be, which is why my dad made the adjustments that were needed to make him, *him*!

The funeral was horrible, hard and overwhelming. I didn't want to say goodbye to a man I loved so much! I remember sitting in the front row with my aunt and her crying on my shoulder through the whole funeral! To this day, it is still one of the hardest things I have ever had to do! During the service we laughed and we cried but mostly we remembered the amazing man who was lying in that casket in front of us!

Watching my uncle's casket carried to the place where he would be forever was heartbreaking. I remember breaking down as they lowered it into the ground, and knowing that I would never see my uncle again. It was the worst feeling in the world! How do you say goodbye to someone who was taken from you far too soon?

*

CHRISTINE BASTONE
Christine's sister Elizabeth
died in 2012 at age 38

My sister Pam, her husband, Paul, and Liz's husband, Adam, planned the memorial service. Since I didn't help plan it, I don't know many of the details. As far as I know, almost everything went smoothly. Or at least as smoothly as could be expected. The only real problem that I know about is that they had a really hard time finding a minister who was willing to speak at the service. Once they found out that Liz had died by suicide, all of them refused. I believe it was a friend of Pam and Paul's who was the minister who ended up speaking. And he was out of town at the time the service was being planned. We had to wait for him to come back to town before we could have the service. This is why we ended up being out of town longer than we had anticipated.

I wasn't there when this was happening. I found out about it about two days before the service. This upset me to no end! How dare they refuse! This only hurts and punishes the family that is left behind. It is not right. Even if Liz deserved that, and I absolutely don't believe that she did, we certainly didn't. Except for the ministers who refused to speak, everybody involved really did an awesome job at planning my sister's memorial service.

Liz's memorial service was very nice. The only things I wish could have been different were that I wasn't ready for it to end, I wish more people would have been there, and that more could have stayed for the get-together afterward.

I got there a half hour early. They were playing a very nice DVD that had a bunch of pictures of Liz with beautiful music playing in the background. I started watching it, and that was the only time that tears came to my eyes that day. It seems that I can cry at anything but funerals and memorial services!

Before it was over, people started coming in. I stopped watching (but got my own copy later), and went to greet them. I was a real social butterfly that day, which is so not like me. I saw people that I hadn't seen in years. That part was nice. Then the service started. It was basically the minister speaking, and then the three eulogies. It's kind of funny, for once I wasn't nervous. Public speaking always makes me nervous, but not that day. Of course I did write out what I was going to say ahead of time, so all I had to do was read it. It was also pretty short. But I think that I did a good job, and I felt like I connected with the audience...so I'm proud of that very important speech.

I was also proud of how well my mother and Pam did as well. And I am happy to say that I have a copy of all of our words to always remember.

After when it was over, people came up to talk to us for just a minute...sort of like a receiving line at a wedding. And then we went to a nearby church for a get-together. A number of people couldn't stay for that. That was disappointing, but I understood. Especially as some of the people only had a day or two of notice. It was so nice of them to come at all. Again I was a social butterfly. I didn't really sit down and eat until I was done talking to everyone. Then we went to Pam's house. My Aunt Barbara, my dad's only sister, came too. We sat down on the couch and talked for a while. She showed us pictures of her kids, my cousins, and their families, and told us all about what was going on with them. I hadn't seen her in I don't know how long, so it was nice to catch up with her. We couldn't stay too late because we were leaving first thing the following morning. So we said our goodbyes and went back to our motel room. It's certainly a day that I will never forget.

*

SHARON EHLERS
Sharon's best friend Joy died in 2009 at age 52,
Sharon's former fiancé John died in 2012 at age 59

Joy's husband and family planned a memorial service for her back in California. I had been given her address book and was asked to call everyone in it. It was so difficult. I had to keep telling the story over and over. Everyone had questions. I had no answers.

I was also asked to give one of the eulogies. I remember sitting in Joy's backyard and writing what came into my head. The tears just flowed and the words poured out. I wanted to remind people about what a kind and loving person Joy was. How she loved holidays and the color pink. How she was one of the best crafts people I knew. How she made a complete bedding set for my youngest daughter's crib out of pink gingham when my daughter was born. I still have that crib bedding set.

Writing that eulogy helped me to heal. The service itself was mostly family, but a few former coworkers were also there. Some had driven quite a distance to pay their respects. Our other best friend, Chris, had flown in from Florida. It was comforting to have her there. Joy, Chris and I were like the Three Musketeers. We had been through a lot together. We had laughed until we cried. We had cried until we laughed. It isn't often that you find two best friends. We were finally together one last time.

When I gave my eulogy, it was hard not to break down, looking at Joy's elderly parents sitting in the front row. They had aged significantly in a short time. Her mom kept asking me why it had happened. I kept telling her I wasn't sure but I knew Joy was tired. Tired of living with sadness. I know that didn't help Joy's mother much, and she died a few months after Joy's death. Probably of a broken heart.

What was sadder to me was that no one seemed to know about or understand the sadness Joy had been experiencing for almost twenty years. How could her family not know? I guess I understood more about Joy in that moment than I ever did. Her desire to make her family proud. To be the perfect daughter. The memorial service was just a reminder to me that Joy kept most of her struggle and pain to herself. She had trusted me enough to share her demons with me, but at that moment, I wasn't sure I felt very honored. In some ways I was angry. Angry that Joy had placed that responsibility on me. Angry that she couldn't be honest. Angry that she didn't get the help she needed. Angry that maybe in some way I had failed her as a friend. Although the memorial service helped us to say goodbye, I had a feeling that this was only the beginning of the pain associated with Joy's death.

After John committed suicide, his family decided to forgo a formal service for him. I understood their decision, but then again I didn't understand. John had friends, and people who loved him. Not paying tribute to him seemed like a slap in his face. John deserved to be remembered; my children and I needed closure. We needed to cry with all the other mourners where it would be appropriate, rather than alone in our car or not at all. It all seemed very confusing. Isn't that what you are supposed to do?

To remedy the lack of a service and to have a chance to share our grief as a family, we decided to have our own. We picked probably one of the most beautiful sunny days here in southern California at a park overlooking the ocean. I read a eulogy I had written. We talked about John's life. We listened to his favorite Beach Boys music. We told stories. We released a balloon. We sat in the park and cried. It didn't matter what the other park-goers thought. This was about us. We needed this. We needed to feel like crap together. After our service was over, my youngest daughter thanked me because she said it had helped her to remember John and share her grief. I knew we had done the right thing by having our own memorial service.

*

BONNIE FORSHEY
Bonnie's son Billy
died in 1993 at age 16

I planned Billy's service with his stepfather. There was a huge group of people who waited in line to pay their respects. They shared their stories with me and sang songs. It was very touching. I never knew that Billy had made such an impact on so many people's lives. The funeral was held the following day at the church we attended. The teens wanted to play "No Tears In Heaven," but the pastor said no. The pastor then started a sermon about suicide and hell. I was appalled, as was everyone else. He told everyone that they should not follow in Billy's footsteps or else they would go to hell. Can you imagine how I felt? I had just lost my son! Our pastor was telling me that Billy was in hell. I left the church and never looked back.

*

LAURA HABEDANK
Laura's brother Brian
died in 2010 at age 35

Having a mother who has worked in a funeral home for as far back as I can recall, I was not at all unfamiliar with the subject of death, funerals or the details that go into planning one. It was all pretty much second nature to me, as I had grown so comfortable with all of it over the years. But accepting the fact that it was now a funeral for my one and only sibling was just unbearable. Nothing about it felt real.

I told my mom that I wanted the opportunity to see my brother's body because I absolutely needed that closure for myself, if only to prove to myself that it was real. I had my mind set on going to the funeral home to view Brian's body. But I never had the chance. The funeral directors, whom I'd known for so many years and consider wonderful friends, came to the house to see me in person and tell me they didn't recommend my seeing him. I recall one of them basically saying to me, "We understand the immense importance of closure, and when at all possible, we give families the chance to see the body of the deceased, even if it means just being able to see a single hand and hold it one last time. I've known Brian for years but in all honesty, if I hadn't been told that it was him, there is no way I'd have recognized him at all. I think it would be detrimental to you to see him in that state and would cause you far more harm than you can imagine." I was devastated. My mind was a blur and my imagination ran absolutely wild. I couldn't control the thoughts racing in my head about how bad Brian must have looked to have been told I couldn't even see a hand or a foot to be able to have that tangible proof for myself. I kept thinking that maybe I should see him because surely the things I'm imagining in my head have to be far worse than reality, you know?

They did take some photos at my request, in case somewhere down the road I change my mind and still feel I need to see them for closure. To be honest, five years later I still have not ruled out asking to see those photos, because I still experience days where a rogue thought gets hold of me and I think, "Maybe this is all just a bad dream. I never did actually see him for myself, so how do I know it was really him?"

For the most part, my mom took care of the details of the funeral. Brian, in his letter to us, had chosen cremation for himself so that's what we did. He wasn't a religious person, nor am I, so we held the service at the funeral home, not in a church. I chose the writings to be included in the funeral program, and my mom and I picked out the songs to be performed together.

The funeral itself was surreal. If only Brian could have seen how deeply he was loved and appreciated — the sheer number of people who showed up to celebrate his life was staggering. I recall one specific moment of the funeral, during one of the songs, when I took a look around the room and felt an overwhelming rush of peace and love as I looked at the sea of faces all there to support me and my family; it's so hard to put into words, but it's as though I felt a collective set of imaginary arms holding me in a warm embrace to let me know I wasn't alone in my grief. It was both heartbreaking and beautiful. It's a moment that has remained as vivid in my memory as the day it happened. I'm so grateful for that feeling.

*

VICKI HECKROTH
Vicki's son Matthew
died in 2000 at age 17

My husband and daughters help me plan Matt's funeral. It tore me apart inside to be picking out a casket, clothes, music, and flowers for my youngest child, my only son. I believe I just put my body on autopilot to get through it all. My ex-husband, Matthew's dad, showed up asking where he should sit at the funeral. He had not seen Matthew since he was three years old; it had been fourteen years. I told him that I really didn't care where he sat. In fact, I didn't care if he was there or not. After the funeral, Matt's dad asked me for half of the memorial money, revealing the real reason he was there. I was instantly beyond angry. And when I was done speaking, he knew he wasn't going to profit off my son's death.

This was one of the worst weeks of my life. The funeral home let us know that after we paid the first three thousand dollars from the memorials we had received, we had one year to pay the remaining twelve thousand dollars. There was no way we had that kind of money, and no life insurance. I felt I had failed my son before his death and then failed him again by having to file for bankruptcy. The funeral home, as well as the lady Matt hit in the auto accident, were both suing us, threatening to take our home. We were left with no choice; it devastated me.

*

MARLISE MAGNA
Marlise's fiancé Blaine
died in 2010 at age 36

A close family friend planned the funeral. Blaine was an only child, and his mother simply couldn't cope. We only met at the morgue, and the entire family was in a state of shock. What stunned me at the funeral was that not only was the family not honest about the cause of death, but also that I was the only one falling to pieces as the hearse drove off. The rest were already sipping on coffee and eating snacks. It made me question the value of our lives to others.

*

MARCELLA MALONE
Marcella's brother Michael
died in 2014 at age 20

Less than twenty-four hours after being notified that Michael had taken his life, we were overwhelmed with questions about when the funeral would be. My mom just opened the phone book and called the first funeral home listed. Twelve hours later, my mom, dad, older brother and his fiancée, and I sat in a room waiting to do the unimaginable. No one had seen this coming, and we struggled to comprehend the reality enough to make decisions. We all wanted it over with.

We chose to have Michael cremated, as my parents wanted to be able to bury him with them. So we had just a simple ceremony at the funeral home. Our friends and family arranged a lunch at our house following it; they were amazing. No urn seemed fit. It wasn't where Michael, so young, belonged. We chose to have his ashes placed in a football. It truly seemed fitting, and was beautiful. The hardest part was probably seeing the obituary in the paper. That's when it really hit home for us that Michael was actually gone.

On April 19, just five days after Michael's death, we prepared for a truly hard day for our family. We lined up at the entrance and everyone offered their love and condolences. Nothing they said seemed right to me and it took everything I had to stay strong. As we moved into the room we had Michael's amazing football coaches as pastors, and his pictures and favorite thing surrounded us. All the seats were filled and people were left standing. The love for Michael was powerful and huge. I just wish he could have seen it. I couldn't leave quick enough when it was over. I was done. That wasn't him. As we returned to our house everything was more relaxed and we honored Michael with food and a party and lots of memory sharing. No drama. That was him and what he deserved. The longest week of my life was over.

*

JULIE MJELVE
Julie's husband Cameron
died in 2011 at age 42

I planned most of the funeral along with my husband's parents. They accompanied me to meet with the funeral director, and we made a lot of the choices together. They were very good at deferring to me for most things but speaking up when they had a strong preference about something. Although things went smoothly and there were no disagreements, it was a difficult experience in a different way. At the time I felt it was my responsibility to plan and organize the funeral, as well as to say the eulogy, since it was my husband who died. However, in looking back, I wish someone would have just done it all for me. I would have preferred to just show up, be the grieving widow and allow myself to be sad, rather than having to participate.

*

GRACE YOUNG
Grace's son Jack
died in 2007 on his 27th birthday

We buried our boy in the cemetery down the road from us. We had to purchase a family plot. We consulted with his brother and Jack's fiancée. Would Jack have wanted to be cremated and have his ashes scattered? Would he have wanted to be buried? His younger brother Ben said, "I don't think Jack would have wanted to be buried in the cold, cold ground." But Jack's fiancée said, "Jack told me if anything ever happened to him, he wanted to be buried with his guitar and leather jacket." And so that is what we did.

It was very difficult to choose a coffin, to see his cold, lifeless body in the funeral parlor morgue. While walking home from the wake after being hugged by so many friends and family, my son Ben said, "You know what, Mom? That was very good." I knew just what he meant. I think Jack would have been surprised that he was loved by so many people. His depression had him thinking that no one loved him. They had asked us if we wanted any special music, and we just could not think of what would have been appropriate. But then I remembered the last song we had figured out how to play on the piano together, "Mad World." So during the burial we played it. Imagine my heartbreak when the lyrics "Children waiting for the day they feel good, happy birthday, happy birthday," came on. I had forgotten those words. I feel bad for the people who had to witness my complete and utter howl of pain when that was played. We had friends and family over to our house afterward, and we all gathered in the backyard. My husband's family all brought food and drinks. We were able to share some sweet memories. My son Ben was a great comfort to us. He helped us greatly.

*

CHAPTER FOUR

THE TRANSITION

The bereaved need more than just the space to grieve the loss. They also need the space to grieve the transition. -LYNDA CHELDELIN FELL

As we begin the transition of facing life without our loved one, some find comfort by immediately returning to a familiar routine, while others find solitude a safe haven. Sometimes our own circumstances don't allow choices to ponder, and we simply follow where the path leads. But the one commonality we're all faced with is the starting point that marks the transition from our old life to the new.

*

KAYLA ARNOLD
Kayla's uncle Tim
died in 2001 at age 34

My sisters and I were out of school a little over a week. I remember it was still so hard to go back to school. Even a week later, I was dealing with emotions, thoughts and feelings that still didn't make any sense to me. I had just buried one of the most important people to me, and still didn't understand how it could be real that he was gone.

As far as my emotions go, I had breakdowns and moments where it was hard but everyone was understanding, supportive, and helped me through it. My sisters, on the other hand, had some rough moments when people were not so understanding. One of my sisters' classmates came up to her and told her that my uncle was going to hell because he killed himself! When my sister said no, he wasn't, the kid said, "Yes, he is. That's what my parents said." My nine-year-old sister had to listen to another nine-year-old tell her my uncle was going to hell because their parents told them that is what would happen. My sister had to feel the pain of that child's harsh words just days after watching our uncle buried.

Thankfully, my parents were part of the school's PTA, and they were able to do some education. They went classroom to classroom and spoke with the students about people not being sinful. They explained to the kids that there is no place in the bible where it says that a person goes to hell. They also talked about reasons why someone might take his life, such as depression and fights. And my parents talked about how hurtful words are, and remembering to be nice to one another because people never know when their words can truly hurt someone.

I am thankful that my uncle's death did come at a time when my parents were able to offer education without a big uproar. It was helpful because, just like my sisters and myself, suicide was not something they knew about, and education is a must when it comes to suicide awareness!

School, work, and sports were hard to go back to. I remember I was doing synchronized swimming for the first time and my performance was just a few weeks after my uncle passed, and he was supposed to be there. That performance was very hard; I can remember looking into the stands, seeing my family and tearing up because he wasn't there. I know he was there in spirit, but it's just not the same when you are missing someone. We returned to our routines, but things were never the same. We were never the same.

*

EMILY BARNHARDT
Emily's friend and roommate Hannah
died in 2014 at age 20

I tried to put off the responsibility of resuming work and college classes as long as I could. The pressure and responsibility felt overwhelming. I was terrified that I wouldn't be able to function and would spiral out of control under the pressure. I simply didn't know how to continue performing and acting like the person I was before Hannah's death.

Simultaneously, I couldn't figure out how the "new" me should act or perform either. I didn't know who I was anymore. In my mind, my experience of trying to jump back into my normal routine and daily life after that devastating loss was like a kid trying to jump mid-swing, yet perfectly synchronized, into a jump rope game.

I was lucky to have a part-time job where my managers were lenient with my schedule after Hannah passed. Come August, however, three months after her death, I had to face the inevitable. I had to resume classes and begin working regularly again. Although the routine was good, I sank into a deep, dull sadness. The shock of trying to process Hannah's death, while also picking up the pieces of her life, kept me moving and functioning in a chaotic yet slow-motion state of being.

It wasn't until those first months passed that fresh grief seemed to settle in my chest and become a dull, permeating ache. On top of my new daily routine that brutally revealed Hannah's absence, I was also adapting to new classes, new people, and a new home after I moved. I found myself looking at a life that was suddenly terrifying and unfamiliar, and I didn't have the slightest clue how to navigate those uncharted waters.

Once I started back at school and work, a friend said to me in conversation, "How are work and school going? You feeling back to normal now?" Words failed me and I felt ashamed, because I was honestly feeling less normal and worse than before. I felt like everyone around me must think I was doing better, simply because I had resumed my daily responsibilities. I sank into isolation, afraid to reveal the ugly truth to those around me that I was lightyears away from feeling anywhere close to normal again.

Being in the usual swing of things, I had hoped I would start to feel like I was moving forward again. But I didn't. And that sent me into panic that I would never move forward; I would forever stay stuck in a state of merely existing. I understand now, however, that the entire concept of "moving forward" is often completely devastating to a grieving person, because after losing someone you so deeply care about, you only want to go backwards. You want to go back to the times when they were alive, when life was familiar, when you could hug them and talk to them.

The superficial conversations at work, school, and within my community of friends were difficult sometimes. I believe that people wanted to engage me in light conversation in an attempt to make me feel more normal, but no amount of pretending could make things feel okay. The superficial conversations, as well intended as they were, only made me feel more isolated. I felt pressured to have interesting, superficial things to say about school, work, life, and volunteer activities. In reality, my daily life consisted of endless crushing reminders, exaggerated by things like having to adjust to a new home that felt strange and unfamiliar, and professors at school unaware that I was sinking under the weight of their expectations. The list was endless. Those superficial conversations that seemed to be the majority of my interactions with people became an unbridgeable chasm and disconnect that separated me from everyone else. It was normal for them to discuss work and school. It wasn't normal for them to discuss me sobbing at the bank, having to explain that I couldn't get my deposit back because Hannah's name was before mine on our check.

I had to give myself the space to grieve more than Hannah's death. I had to let myself grieve the change, the transition, the distance from my friends. I had to grieve losing the life I had known and grieve the little pieces of Hannah I lost every time something new came up unexpectedly.

The transition was tougher for me than the immediate aftermath when shock shielded me from full comprehension of the loss. In the transition, shock abandoned me, somewhat stripping me of its protection. I was then forced to start facing reality at whatever pace it came each day. It can be tough for the bereaved when outsiders don't understand this. It's understandable how most people assume that the immediate aftermath of the loss is the most excruciating time period. Though it certainly is excruciating and tumultuous, the ensuing transition is equally agonizing. And it would ease the loneliness and difficulty, whether little or tremendously, if we could teach and help those who support us to better understand that.

*

CHRISTINE BASTONE
Christine's sister Elizabeth
died in 2012 at age 38

I don't have a paying job, I'm a stay-at-home mom. We were out of town for about a week; that's how long my husband took off of work, and also how long I pulled my kids out of school. The transition went smoothly for my husband and my kids. For those first few months it was very hard for me to focus even on basic things, such as getting my kids off to school and making dinner every night. I was grieving pretty close to twenty-four hours a day at that point. Focusing on anything else was extremely difficult. I did the best I could but I was relieved when summer came, and I didn't have to get the kids to and from school for a few months.

*

SHARON EHLERS
Sharon's best friend Joy died in 2009 at age 52,
Sharon's former fiancé John died in 2012 at age 59

Joy died on a Sunday. I went to work on Monday. Or let's say I tried to work on Monday. I went to work because I couldn't face being home alone with time to think. Once I got to work, though, I realized it was a mistake. I sat at my desk and stared at the computer screen. I couldn't have gotten anything done if someone had paid me a million dollars to do it. I eventually went home after a couple of hours. As I think about it now, one of the reasons work was twice as hard that day was because I walked in to find a voicemail from my former fiancé, John, who had heard about Joy's death. He knew Joy too, and knew how close we were. John offered his condolences. It touched my heart, because I hadn't heard from him in a while. It made me more emotional than I was when I walked in. Needless to say, I went home and made plans for the drive to Las Vegas. I had never made the five-hour trip alone, but it didn't matter. I needed the time alone in the car to cry. I got there in one piece and stayed until the following Sunday. I left Las Vegas one week to the day after Joy's death. I felt like a piece of me stayed there with her. After driving the usual eight-hour trip in Sunday traffic from Las Vegas to Los Angeles, I somehow made it in to work the next day. My head still wasn't together.

I don't know how I made it through those first weeks. I just struggled through it like everyone does. I bought books on suicide, thinking I might find some answers. I walked outside as much as I could so I could cry in private. I prayed as much as I could. I talked to Joy as much as I could. I asked my Reiki teacher for a Reiki session to help me calm down and relax. It helped tremendously. Most important, I spoke with Joy as much as I could and asked her to send me signs. The signs were what kept me going. They helped me to transition back into the land of the living. Work was still hard, but the pain was not debilitating.

After John's death I did not take any time off. I went right back to work. I should have learned after Joy's death that this doesn't work. I guess I needed a second life lesson. After John's death it didn't work either. Especially difficult were the phone calls I got at work after his death, like the detective who was working John's case, and John's mom. Thank God I had a door to my office. I just kept it closed. One day it was so tough that I told my boss what was going on. He was so understanding. He suggested I leave early that day and I did, gratefully.

People just didn't know what to say to me. In fact, many avoided talking to me. I don't think it was their fault, I just think they didn't know what to say. Our society isn't very good at dealing with suicide. And when you are on the work front, you have to put up that fake smile and pretend everything is okay. Many coworkers probably have no idea to this day what happened with John.

I really tried to make sure that when I wasn't at work I grieved as much as I could. I hit grief head-on. I forced myself to look at old pictures. To go through the box of "memories" I had saved. I listened to the music that was a part of our relationship. I read old letters out loud in the hopes that he could hear what I had written.

I also joined a Survivors After Suicide support group. I had looked into it after Joy's death, but never did it. I figured after John died that I had no excuse. It was now or never. It was a great relief to be with a group of people who had similar (or worse) experiences. It was a relief to not have to hide. It was a relief to talk about it.

I think that forcing myself to grieve helped me get through those days at work, and life in general, in a better frame of mind. It didn't make the sadness go away but it gave me an outlet for all my emotions. And from what I could tell, that was a good thing.

*

BONNIE FORSHEY
Bonnie's son Billy
died in 1993 at age 16

I went back to work about six months later, but couldn't deal with it. The high school was right next door, and I could look out the window and see Billy's friends going on with their lives. I found another position in a different town, and worked many hours trying to block out the ghosts.

*

LAURA HABEDANK
Laura's brother Brian
died in 2010 at age 35

I had been at my new job only for thirty days when Brian died, so I had very little support at my new job; I really didn't know anyone there very well yet. I came back to work only eleven days after getting the news of Brian's death, so in only ten days I had flown home from Texas to Minnesota, helped plan his funeral, cleaned out his home of all his belongings, suffered through his funeral and the empty days afterward, and then flew back to Texas to get back to "real life" again.

I recall getting to work early that Monday, feeling sick to my stomach, as I knew I absolutely was not feeling even remotely ready to get back to reality. As I sat down to turn on my computer, my manager bounced past me with a huge smile and said, "Hey,

Laura! Good morning!! How are you??" But I guess that was more of a rhetorical question anyway, as she kept walking and didn't stick around for an answer. My heart hit the floor. That was the kind of greeting you give someone who has just returned from vacation, not someone returning from the funeral of her only sibling who just died by suicide. I began to sob quietly at my desk, and thought how I had never felt so alone in my life. My pain wasn't acknowledged, and that hurt a great deal but I found out the hard way that people don't want to deal with things that make them uncomfortable, so they just don't.

For the most part, I was avoided completely by my new coworkers, and few people even looked me in the eye. Not a single person said so much as, "I'm sorry for your loss." It was one of the most lonely and alienating experiences of my life.

Having been at the job for only a month so far, I was still in training, and I found myself struggling in the most unimaginable way. Not only was I feeling depressed, lonely and suicidal, but I was desperately trying to take in loads of new information for which I was going to be responsible while I was suffering from a complete and total lack of focus. My mind was elsewhere, and I had loads of trouble trying to process the things I was being taught. Information was going in and right back out again, so on top of feeling sad I was also feeling panicked that I was going to be fired because I just wasn't "catching on" and wasn't pulling my weight on the team. I absolutely dreaded going into work each day, and usually all the way to work, during my bathroom breaks, during my lunch hour, and on the drive home. For the most part I was able to hold back the tears when others were watching. But, there were times when I just didn't care who saw me crying, because it didn't really matter… it's not as though anyone seemed to care, anyway. You can cry all you want when you're invisible.

A month after the funeral, the manager at the company I'd left for this new job contacted me and asked if I would come back to work for them. She had heard from a mutual friend that I was struggling, and she offered me the chance to come back to work and again be surrounded by people who cared for me. I jumped at the chance. I'm still there five years later, and honestly, I'm grateful for that gesture every single day. The magnitude and importance of what that did for me is not lost on me. Everyone here welcomed me back with open arms and hugs and listening ears. Even if they didn't understand, they cared enough to try.

*

VICKI HECKROTH
Vicki's son Matthew
died in 2000 at age 17

I returned to work three days after the funeral. It was the worst thing I could have done. Matthew had worked there with me, so he was missing when I was home and also when I was at work. I was a waitress, and the customers all knew me, so of course the questions and condolences were abundant. I spent much time in the restroom crying. My husband also returned to work that day. He is in an auto body shop and pretty much works by himself, so it wasn't as hard on him. It actually gave him something to keep his mind off things.

My oldest daughter was pregnant with twins, so she didn't work. Her husband told her not to get sad because it wasn't good for the babies, so she shouldn't think about it. She had a really hard time having to hide her mourning. My middle daughter had a baby girl five months old and also did not work. She had a hard time with guilt because Matt had wanted to spend the weekend with her, but her significant other had said no. She felt that had Matt been with her, he would still have been alive. But we all know this was not her fault. My entire family had such a hard time, and still do at times. My father told me this was my fault. He said that had

I been a better mother and home with Matt instead of working, he would still be here. I wasn't working because I wanted to, but because I had to. And Matt was seventeen. He was either working or out and about himself. I will never have a close relationship with my father because of his words to me. Many people blamed us as parents, saying there must have been something wrong in our home life for Matt to have done this. Many friends left because they didn't want to hear about it any longer, and all I wanted to do was talk about it. I still do. Because talking about my son and saying his name keeps his memories alive. He lived, and he matters. We were shunned, talked about. People acted as if they could catch suicide from us. Our lives went from good to bad in just that instant.

*

MARLISE MAGNA
Marlise's fiancé Blaine
died in 2010 at age 36

I never really returned to work fully after the ordeal. My entire life spun out of control, and I lived not even day to day but hour to hour. It's embarrassing to say now, but for a few weeks I became a total hermit, lived off alcohol and medication, sitting in front of the TV in a state of suspended disbelief. I couldn't even bring myself to bathe, brush my hair or change my clothes. I was a hot mess. To this day I do only freelance work.

About two years after Blaine passed, I became born again and am currently in ministry. That has given me some peace but I am still very anxious and scared to commit to this day. I am very fortunate that my family, my mom especially, have all been very supportive, both financially and emotionally. I am also surrounded by an awesome support structure of friends.

*

MARCELLA MALONE
Marcella's brother Michael
died in 2014 at age 20

Everyone returned to work and school at their own pace. It took my parents over a month, and it was still rough on them. My brother and his fiancée had to return to work the following week. For me, that week was the start of final papers and projects being turned in and/or presented and exams being taken. I had a lot to catch up on, and no choice but to return to school the Monday following the funeral. It wasn't as easy as it sounded. I struggled to concentrate on anything other than what I had lost. I ended up failing half of my classes that semester. It was rough on me, and knocked me out of the running for future grad school plans.

Little did I know at the time that I would find a much better fit shortly after, a field that could help other kids from making the same decision my brother did. My boss was very understanding and told me to come back to work when I was ready. It was hard having free time to sit at home and think about the past and future. I ended up returning to work that Friday. My coworkers were great about working with me to provide support and a break when I was having a weak moment. I will always be thankful for that.

*

BRIDGET PARK
Bridget's brother Austin
died in 2008 at age 14

I returned to school about three weeks after the suicide of my brother Austin. It was a few days before my thirteenth birthday. I purposely was late to my first class, and I will never forget walking into the classroom and everyone turning their heads toward me.

Everyone knew my brother and was fully aware of what happened, because we lived in a small town. Also, everyone from my school knew about my brother's suicide because my middle school and my brother's high school were together in one building.

I was extremely nervous about returning to school, because someone at my school started a rumor that I had gotten in a fight with Austin and then I shot him. That rumor hurt and disgusted me more than I can ever put into words. But when I returned to school my peers were very sympathetic, thankfully, and the rumor never came up.

From then on my peers were really supportive, but sometimes the way they tried to support me had the opposite effect. Girls came forward saying that he was "like a brother to me," and it was very hurtful for me to hear that. I felt like people were acting like they knew my brother well so they could get attention from others, whereas I did everything in my power to seem somewhat stable and trying to hide my pain. I kept to myself and communicated with my two best friends only when at school. I steered away from other students and friends because I knew that my presence made them uneasy. I felt like an animal in a glass box that everyone stared at in awe, like I was a rare species.

My school, however, was very supportive and more than willing to provide whatever tools were necessary for me to catch up in school and to receive proper help. The teachers were understanding when I skipped class to be alone and cry. They understood when I would get up and leave in the middle of class. But after I had my time alone, I would be called in to speak to the counselors. I was blessed to have such understanding teachers.

*

GRACE YOUNG
Grace's son Jack died
in 2007 on his 27th birthday

I was out of work for two weeks. We needed that time to retrieve Jack's things and make the arrangements. It was also the maximum my employer allowed for the death of a child. Personally, I think employers should allow more time for a suicide death. Everyone treated me differently; they really didn't know what to say, and they just didn't talk to me much. I was pleased that my boss and coworkers came to the wake and funeral, but after two weeks it was like "Oh, well, business as usual." Customers who knew me well also did not want to discuss my loss, and everyone just kind of looked at me with pity. It was very hard to go back to work, and I wish I didn't have to.

*

CHAPTER FIVE

THE QUESTION

Grievers use a very simple calendar. Before and after. -LYNDA CHELDELIN FELL

One day we have our loved one, the next day he or she is no longer a living possibility. How do we explain to others something we can't wrap our brain around? How do we answer the question "How did your loved one die?"

*

KAYLA ARNOLD
Kayla's uncle Tim
died in 2001 at age 34

When answering that question, I am very straightforward. I will either say that Uncle Tim committed suicide, or that he took his own life. If they then ask me how he did it, I am honest and tell them that he shot himself. And if they ask where, I tell them that he shot himself in his head. If they ask whether Uncle Tim passed away quickly, I explain that the bullet killed him instantly. I firmly believe in being honest and straightforward when it comes to my uncle's death, because if they ask questions and I am able to educate someone on suicide and suicide prevention, I will do it gladly!

When Uncle Tim first passed away, I found it very hard to talk about it and would tear up or cry when talking about him and how he died. But over time it's become a way for me to educate and help others, and I look at it as a way that something good could come from losing my uncle!

*

EMILY BARNHARDT
Emily's friend and roommate Hannah
died in 2014 at age 20

For a period of time, I wrestled a lot over how to respond when people asked me how Hannah died. It wasn't from my own uncertainty, rather it was from the opinions I have sensed from others at times. Suicide is often a stigmatized and taboo subject, and after the first two months of her passing, there were moments when it felt like she had become a taboo subject as well.

In some conversations I noticed that whenever I mentioned Hannah's name, even lightly in reference to a funny memory or something I was currently doing, it was as if the air around the conversation became instantly thin. Some people wouldn't acknowledge the mention of her name at all, while others might give a nod of acknowledgment and a smile before changing the subject. It felt very uncomfortable sometimes. I wanted people to understand that if I ever brought Hannah up it was because I wanted to, which meant it was okay for them to talk about her, too. It meant I was okay with it and wanted to be able to mention her. It still is this way. It isn't this way for every person grieving, but I find comfort in mentioning or talking about Hannah. I want to say her name and share stories. If it's a situation where I would mention her if she were alive, then I refuse to not mention her now just because she's gone. It comforts me, because it allows me to acknowledge that she did, and still does, matter deeply to me.

When people ask how Hannah died, I'm honest. I say that she took her own life, because I don't want her memory to become taboo simply because of the stigma around suicide. There are usually always feelings of anxiety when I answer though. I wonder what that person might think about me…was I not a good friend? Did I love Hannah well, or was I selfish and oblivious to her pain? How could I have let that happen? Did I even try to help her?

In reality, I have no idea if these thoughts ever actually cross anyone's mind. Perhaps that insecurity merely indicates that I still wrestle with those questions myself. I've thought a lot about why there is hesitancy when it comes to sharing that a loved one died by suicide. I think it's the stigma around it. I don't want to be ashamed of or insecure about how Hannah died. I have no reason to be, because the way she died doesn't define her. The Hannah I knew and loved is not the Hannah who took her life. Her actions that night were in response to an impulsive moment of blind pain that consumed her. She saw no other way out, and I don't think less of her for that, and I don't want anyone else to either.

One of my biggest hesitations in being honest about how Hannah died is due to the common responses I've experienced from people shaking their heads in disappointment and commenting on how selfish suicide is. Hearing this response from others is probably the most significant factor that makes me uneasy sharing the truth, because it hurts me deeply when people say things like that. It feels disrespectful to the person Hannah was and disrespectful of my love for her.

I understand why people say suicide is selfish; it's a choice made that hurts others. But in my mind, the word "choice" isn't always an applicable word in the circumstance of suicide. "Choice" implies that a person is able to rationally make a decision about something. Suicide is anything but rational, and no one can judge another's actions without experiencing their state of mind, their pain, their fear, and their despair in that moment.

Hannah had stopped taking her medication – a medication that altered the chemistry of her brain. When you abruptly stop taking a brain-altering medication, the sudden drop in the level of neuro-transmitters from that medication can cause your brain to go haywire. I hurt deeply for Hannah - for what she must have been feeling that night and for how her brain might have been functioning irrationally.

If someone makes a comment about Hannah's death being selfish, it translates to me that her level of pain, and the person she truly was, isn't significant enough to factor into their opinion of Hannah and what happened. So though I generally choose to tell the truth, there are certain situations when I don't if I fear getting responses like these. While I choose to tell the truth, that in no way makes me think differently of those who choose not to.

The most important truth of grief is that everyone grieves differently, and no specific way of grieving is right or wrong. The emotions of grief are universal, but the experience of grief is not. Grief is individual to each person based on his or her own unique personality and methods of coping with trauma. We should expect diverse responses in processing a loss like this, because there are different variables to each person's grief process, due to different factors in our loss and the type of relationship we had with our loved one. No single person's grief can possibly be identical to another's.

Some people find comfort in telling the truth and in talking about their loved one often, while others cope better by maintaining a boundary of privacy around their grief. No response is better than the other, so allow yourself to grieve the way you need to. This grieving and healing journey is yours alone, and you have every right to approach it in the way that will be healthiest and most comforting to you. Only you know what that approach is, so honor that. Honor your limits and your boundaries.

*

CHRISTINE BASTONE
Christine's sister Elizabeth
died in 2012 at age 38

I am speaking only for myself here, but I always say that my sister died by suicide. I am not ashamed of that fact. I am also not at all interested in trying to hide it. And fortunately no one in my family wanted to try to hide it either. Thankfully I don't have any trouble saying the word "suicide." Not that I say it casually or lightly, you understand. I've just said it a lot over the last three years!

I also believe that suicide thrives in silence, so I speak up on the subject. And one of the ways I do that is to say that Liz died by suicide. In fact, I am incredibly grateful that I don't live in a time where suicide is a much more taboo subject and is spoken of in whispers, if it's even spoken of at all. This would be infinitely harder for me to deal with if I couldn't talk about it, including mentioning that my loved one died by suicide!

*

SHARON EHLERS
Sharon's best friend Joy died in 2009 at age 52
Sharon's former fiancé John died in 2012 at age 59

When someone asks about how either Joy or John died, I have always answered with the truth. They committed suicide. It's been my experience that very few people want to know the dreaded "how," so I never say it unless they ask. For the very few (and there haven't been many) who are interested or just morbidly curious, I tell them that both Joy and John put a gun to his or her head and pulled the trigger. Joy did it outside in the backyard by the bathroom window by the side of the house. The bullet went through her head, through the window, and lodged inside the bathroom wall. John sat in the chair I had bought him when we were together, put two pillows over each side of his head, and then pulled the trigger. When they found him the next morning, he was still alive so they flew him by Medevac to the local trauma center. He died there. So there you have it. The raw details.

Personally, I don't think the details should matter. Most people don't know what to say anyway once you have said "suicide." Usually I get "I'm sorry," and then they change the subject. Very few people have wanted to hear or have allowed me to talk about it. That's fine. It's a tough subject anyway. That's why I sought out the Survivors After Suicide support group. Talking about it there gave me the comfort and support I needed. There was no stigma, no funny looks, no one changing the subject.

To this day I always tear up when I talk about their suicides. There is so much emotion attached to their being gone that I typically choke up. But I am not embarrassed or feel like I have to hide it. Life is tough. People have a hard time navigating its twists and turns. Some people have a harder time than others and decide to give up. It's their choice. There was nothing I could have done to stop it. I am at peace with that now. What matters is how they lived. People tend to forget about that. They focus on how it happened. The fact that they committed suicide shouldn't define Joy and John. It's how they lived their lives that is their true legacy.

*

BONNIE FORSHEY
Bonnie's son Billy
died in 1993 at age 16

My son ended his life by an intentional overdose of prescription medications. Obviously something was making him unhappy, although I had no clue. He kept it well hidden from me and always wore a smile.

*

LAURA HABEDANK
Laura's brother Brian
died in 2010 at age 35

I've never shied away from the truth about Brian's death, because there is nothing to be ashamed of. I have always felt that he died from depression just as some people die from cancer or a heart attack. In my opinion, not being honest about it only serves to perpetuate the stigma around depression, mental illness and suicide. It may seem selfish, but I don't tailor my answer to my audience. Unless it's a child who asks me how my brother died, I just tell them he was very sick and died from his illness. It's true, but doesn't force them to hear something that developmentally they may not be ready to hear.

But as far as adults are concerned, I don't ever hold back to make others more comfortable. The reactions I receive from people are so varied; some people become noticeably uncomfortable and change the subject. Some people just sort of stop in their tracks with a blank stare on their faces as words fail them. But the most wonderful responses have been from those who don't allow that to become an awkward moment, because it doesn't need to be. I recall one acquaintance who simply said, "I'm so sorry for your loss. Tell me about your brother, what was he like?" Giving me that little bit of empathy and allowing me to share some memories of Brian was so unbelievably kind and loving; I'm so grateful for that, and wish more people responded that way.

It's been shocking, the number of people we called close friends or family who have "disappeared" from our lives. It seems that when people don't know what to say or do, they just remove themselves from the equation altogether. It's hard not to internalize that and accept that it has more to do with their inability to deal with a painful reality than it does with me. A death by suicide is definitely more alienating, I believe. There are always going to be individuals who will be judgmental about it and feel that sympathy isn't deserved when the person chose his or her own death.

*

VICKI HECKROTH
Vicki's son Matthew
died in 2000 at age 17

My son, Matthew, died by a self-inflicted gunshot wound to the head. He knew just how to aim the shotgun to kill himself instantly. He was seventeen and a junior in high school.

*

MARLISE MAGNA
Marlise's fiancé Blaine
died in 2010 at age 36

I believe honesty is best. I'm not Willy Wonka, so I don't sugarcoat things. I just openly admit that Blaine committed suicide. His family, however, chose to tell people he suffered a heart attack. I guess it was too shameful for them to admit.

*

MARCELLA MALONE
Marcella's brother Michael
died in 2014 at age 20

A year and a half later and still in shock over the loss of my brother, I can honestly admit I dread being asked how it happened. Each day I struggle over the harsh reality of his choice and do my best to suppress the many unanswerable questions that fill my head. Still, it is a big part of my life and a question I am faced with frequently. Common small talk leads most people to ask about your family and siblings. When asked about how many siblings I have, I always include Michael, as we were so close and it simply comes so naturally, but I also mention that he is no longer here. Instinctually it leads to what everyone has to say: "I'm so sorry, what happened?" Because of how strongly the way in which Michael left this earth affected my family and me, for most people I reply with a simple "He took his life." How much more info I give on the happenings of that day depend on how well I know the individual or if they knew my brother. Honestly, those details aren't everyone's business, and too frequently bring out a weak side of me that I don't want everyone to see. The look of pity and/or sadness on people's faces when I talk about it is sometimes too much for me. I want to talk about my brother and his impact, but I don't want that one action to define him or me or anyone else in my family. At the end of the day, I believe it is always best to tell the truth about Michael's passing; suicide is too taboo for how common it is, and I want people to be comfortable talking about it with me. My only exception to this is small children. I tell them that Michael died in his car. It's too much to explain to such an innocent life.

*

JULIE MJELVE
Julie's husband Cameron
died in 2011 at age 42

How I answer the question "How did your loved one die?" depends on who I'm talking to. If it's not someone I trust with the information, or someone I'm speaking to just in person, I often just say, "He was sick," referring to the mental health portion as the cause of Cameron's death. It's still always like a knife in my stomach having to tell new people that he's even dead, let alone the cause. So I've learned to really choose my moments carefully and filter what I reveal. There are some moments now where I do feel

81

it's appropriate to immediately reveal that it was suicide, but for the most part I find it's often not necessary for the conversation.

Also, I find that although I'm able to talk about it, not everyone is in a place to receive it. It especially seems that in this day and age people are expecting the answer to be 'cancer', and when it's not they're thrown because they aren't prepared to deal with suicide. So as I said, I've learned to judge the situation and the person before I decide just how much information is necessary and appropriate.

*

BRIDGET PARK
Bridget's brother Austin
died in 2008 at age 14

My older brother passed away in 2008 due to suicide. Never in a million years would anyone think that my brother would do such a thing. He was popular, handsome, intelligent, and well liked by everyone. So when someone asks me, "How did your brother die?" I have to brace myself for their reaction, because it may be sympathetic or even judgmental. If I do not feel comfortable with this person, or I likely won't see them again, I lie and say that my brother got sick or was in a car accident. But if I know that lying is not the best solution for a particular situation, I will be honest but immediately defend my brother and say that he never showed any signs, and that he was a happy person but just made a knee-jerk decision. It is just easier this way, because I don't have to feel like I am being judged, or my brother too. It is then pretty risk-free overall.

In spite of this, I have learned to not be ashamed or scared of my past, or to hide it from others. As painful or awkward as it can be to tell someone that my brother shot himself, I have learned that each time those words leave my mouth, the less painful it becomes.

*

GRACE YOUNG
Grace's son Jack died
in 2007 on his 27th birthday

Yes, I do tell people that my son died by suicide. It's important to me that people know how easily depression can take over. I say, "My firstborn son, Jack Young Jr., died by suicide on his twenty-seventh birthday, May 8, 2007. We formed Particle Accelerator, in memory of Jack Young Jr., an annual music festival in Putnam, Connecticut, to bring families together in a fun picnic atmosphere to teach them the signs of depression and suicide." It seems that when I feel compelled to share my son's story, it's always to a person who has had a suicide loss. In the eight years that have passed since Jack's death, my reaction is pretty much the same. I have to be bold, to speak up and share his life in order to SAVE a life, no matter how much it hurts.

*

JUST YESTERDAY
BY LYNDA CHELDELIN FELL

Tomorrow is your birthday.
But just yesterday I could hear your voice,
smell your hair, touch your skin.
It's been five years, but the pain still runs deep.
So very, very deep.

They say the pain changes with time. It hasn't.
But I have. My coping skills are stronger. I am stronger.
I like to think I'm a better person with more compassion,
more awareness of the world outside my own.
But the pain runs deep.
So very, very deep.

The tears still fall, and from time to time
I need to retreat to The Wailing Tent
where I'm among sisters. I suppose I always will.
For the pain runs deep.
So very, very deep.

But most days the sun shines bright, and I am grateful.
Today is not one of those days, though.
I want to tell you happy birthday, but the words just won't come.
I know I'm a few hours early anyway,
so maybe the words will come tomorrow.
Oh, the pain runs deep.
So very, very deep.

It feels like yesterday that I could hear your voice,
smell your hair, and touch your skin.
I wish it were yesterday.

*

CHAPTER SIX

THE DATES

No matter what anyone says about grief and about time healing all wounds, the truth is, there are certain sorrows that never fade away until the heart stops beating and the last breath is taken.
-UNKNOWN

Our expectations and memories of balloons and cakes and presents are as regular as the rising sun. When our loved one dies by suicide, how do we acknowledge the painful date they were born, and the date that marks when he or she took his or her own life?

*

KAYLA ARNOLD
Kayla's uncle Tim
died in 2001 at age 34

The anniversary of my uncle's death is by far the hardest. Over time it has gotten a little easier to function on that day, but it is still hard! When he first passed I would spend a lot of the day crying, very sad and simply emotionally drained. With time it has gotten a little easier to not be so upset. Sometimes there are tears but mostly it's just a day where I feel off. Sometimes I'm grumpy, sometimes there is a simple gloominess to my day, but it's functional now, because in the beginning there was not a day that was functional.

I usually post some pictures of Uncle Tim on social media and talk about him and how I miss him. Depending on what I have to do for the day, sometimes I talk about him, just telling stories and remembering him! I find that remembering the good times makes it easier. No matter how hard that day is, looking at pictures and remembering the amazing man he was makes it easier!

The anniversary of Uncle Tim's death is the hardest day. For his birthday and other holidays, I simply remember him and the memories I have of him.

*

EMILY BARNHARDT
Emily's friend and roommate Hannah
died in 2014 at age 20

I've passed the one-year mark since Hannah's death. It's a victory to know that I survived the "year of firsts," as they say. I'm not naïve enough to think, however that the years to come won't still bring up new grief or painful emotions.

Hannah's birthday this year was devastating for me. I felt distant from many of my friends and support system, so I was too afraid to ask for help. I thought I could tough it out on my own by being alone all day. Hannah and I used to regularly have what we called "date nights," where we would go out to dinner and do a fun activity, just the two of us. We cherished that time together. Though we already spent so much time together at home, doing errands, taking classes together, getting our nails done or grabbing lunch, there was something meaningful to us in intentionally planning a special night just for us.

There was a Mexican restaurant that we loved and went to together all the time. On her birthday this year, Hannah's first birthday after her death, I went to that restaurant alone. We'd gone there to celebrate her birthday the previous two years, and I felt the need to go there in honor of her. I thought I would be okay going by myself, but as I sat at that table for one, looking at the empty chair and the place setting across from me that the server had forgotten to clear away, I was overcome with the reality of her absence. I could see her image sitting there, smiling and laughing, and it broke my heart.

Our birthdays were only fourteen days apart, and I was surprised to find that my own birthday was immensely more painful to me than hers was. Because of the season of deep loneliness I felt, due to the distance my grief had put between me and my community of friends, I didn't even mention my upcoming birthday to people. I didn't plan anything to celebrate. I regret that now, because spending most of my birthday alone was extremely difficult. All I could think of was my birthday the previous year when Hannah tackled me in my bed that morning, holding presents and singing to me. I thought back to the year before that when she woke me up for breakfast with a cake she had baked herself. I remembered laughing over how the candles spelling "Happy Birthday" were already melted beyond recognition. I had laughed even harder when she played a video of robots singing "Happy Birthday" to me as she danced along with it. Being without her on my birthday made me realize just how deeply she had always made me feel loved and special and celebrated. So as I sat alone in my quiet apartment on my birthday, her absence was all I could feel and all I could think about.

The anniversary of Hannah's death was easier than I expected, though not easy in the slightest. I again went to the Mexican restaurant we loved, but this time I took a close friend with me. I went out to dinner with two other dear friends.

Later that night Hannah's parents flew down to Florida to be with me, Hannah's boyfriend and some other friends she had loved, and to revisit the place where her life had thrived. I cherish having been able to spend that night with them. We held a small memorial in a gazebo by the Intracoastal Waterway with a beautiful picture of Hannah surrounded by candles at the front. We took turns sharing about her: what we loved about her, how she touched our lives, and what we've learned or realized since her death. We attempted to set off Chinese lanterns in her honor, but the sprinkles of rain coming down made each lantern burst into flames and crumple to the ground in little fireballs. It's a beautiful memory for me though, because we found so much joy and laughter in that, knowing how hard Hannah would have laughed. She would have thought it was hilarious and I could hear the sound of her laughter in my memory. I remember the comfort I felt as we all stood in the rain, laughing at our flaming lanterns crashing to the ground. Hannah would have wanted us to laugh. She loved finding humor in everything.

Looking back, I know I should have reached out for support on our birthdays, and I also wish I had done something to honor her while receiving that support. People always suggest doing something like sending up a balloon into the sky, or writing a letter, or something similar. I thought about doing something like that on those anniversaries, but I couldn't get myself to do it. I just wasn't ready. At first I felt guilty; how could I not do something special to honor her? But I gave myself the gift of compassion, knowing that I just wasn't ready yet, and that it was okay.

For a while, the complicated emotions from how Hannah died made it hard for me to think of her in a peaceful and comforting way, because all I could think of was the despair and darkness she felt that had led her to take her own life. At that time, the idea of doing something peaceful to honor her conflicted with my heart's deep turmoil over her death. It didn't mean I loved her any less; I just hadn't reached a place of stillness where I could do that yet.

I plan to find something special to do to honor Hannah on her birthday and on the anniversary of her death in the years to come. I also know I need to reach out for support when I need it. Maybe what I choose to do in her honor will be something I do every year, or maybe I will allow it to change based on what that specific year has been like for me. I don't know yet, and I'm okay with that. There's no pressure; I will cross that bridge when I come to it.

*

CHRISTINE BASTONE

Christine's sister Elizabeth

died in 2012 at age 38

For my sister's birthday, I bake frosted brownies as a kind of cake. Then I invite my parents over. We light one candle and put it on the cake, and then put the cake in the middle of my kitchen table. We sing "Happy Birthday" while my son records us, and later he uploads it to YouTube. And of course we all eat a piece of her cake.

I also donate to my local library a book that's dedicated in her memory, as a sort of gift to my sister. This is always something on the subject of suicide, or is somehow related to the subject of suicide. For Liz's first birthday after she died, I cooked a dinner that she would have liked, and I also hosted a Facebook event for her. That was a bit much to do again, though. So now I just do the cake and the gift.

The one thing that I didn't expect was how difficult my birthday was. That definitely took me by surprise! I expected Liz's birthday to be difficult. But that wasn't too bad. Maybe because I am still able to do things to observe the day, and honor her. But on my birthday, the thing that I want the most is a card from my baby sister. And unfortunately that is the one thing that I cannot have.

For my sister's death anniversary, I host a Facebook event. I've made it to be like an online memorial service. There are pictures of flowers, there are YouTube videos, there is something that I've written for the occasion such as an updated eulogy. There is also a slideshow. There are a few videos of me playing handbell solos.

There are pictures with pretty online frames, and there are colleges. I work on it little by little all year. A lot of times I work on it on the tenth of the month; those are the "monthaversary" days. It not only keeps me busy, but it also gives me something very important to do on those anniversary days I'm sure would be so much more difficult to deal with if I didn't do something like that.

*

SHARON EHLERS

Sharon's best friend Joy died in 2009 at age 52
Sharon's former fiancé John died in 2012 at age 59

March 3 is Joy's birthday. Since she died, I have still tried to remember her birthday every year. I am sure there are some people who think that is weird or morbid. Personally, I think it is healthy and honest. Joy was my best friend for many years so remembering her just seems like the right thing to do.

I don't dwell on the fact that she isn't here anymore. I don't dwell on how and why she died. I just focus on all the great memories we had together. The last birthday I spent with Joy was her fiftieth birthday party. She was in her element. Joyful (no pun intended) and so happy that all her friends and family were around her on her special day. She told me that she felt that day was the best day of her life. She loved being reminded how much she meant to everyone. Don't we all need that? Being reminded that we mean something to someone else? Joy reveled in it that day.

Joy meant everything to me. Words can't come close to describing the feeling. I think this framed saying I gave to her, and was able to keep after her death, may come close: One of the greatest blessings in my life is our friendship. When I need to talk, you are there to "just listen." You are the person I can laugh with about the most important life events. You "know me" and that saves words sometimes. Thank you for sharing your friendship with me. You are my best friend.

I also remember the anniversary of Joy's death every year. October 11, her grief anniversary. I think it is important to do this. I want Joy to know I haven't forgotten her. I usually wear pink, because she loved it so much. Sometimes I will walk around Wal-Mart, which was her favorite store. I know she is there with me walking up and down the aisles. I want to celebrate Joy and her life here on earth. She deserved that much.

I always call John's mom on his birthday and grief anniversary. Since time does not heal when it comes to grief, it is not surprising that the grief anniversary of John's death is just as painful as the day he died. The pain of his death has been soul-wrenching and gut-stomping. Time couldn't possibly ever heal that wound. Why would I want it to?

Since John died on April 3, the third of every month that first year became a recurring, in-your-face reminder that he was gone. It's been two months. It's been five months. It's been nine months. So I decided that I had two choices about how I was going to handle it: bottle it all up inside and walk around pretending I was okay, or face it head-on and let the emotions flow. So on the third (and most other days), I spent the time crying until there were no tears left. I shouted at the sky. I took long walks. I went through old pictures. I read old cards and love letters. I listened to "our" songs. I remembered the good and the bad. I called his mom and we cried together. I had a memorial service for him with my children up on a hill overlooking the ocean, and we released a balloon to the heavens. We cried and held each other. I just let it all out. Then I let it out some more until I felt empty. The emptiness didn't lessen the sadness or the pain, but it felt better than holding it inside.

On his grief anniversary, I wanted it to be about him and the joy he brought to my life. The laughter. The great memories. The soul-embracing love. Pizza and margaritas. Hawaiian sunsets. Las Vegas fun. The U.S. Open in New York. Boat rides on Lake Anna. Crawling out a window to shovel snow on the deck. The "Aflac" duck commercials. John Wayne. The Beach Boys. I released another balloon on the hill overlooking the ocean. I listened to at least one of "our" songs one more time. It's important to have this time, no matter how sad it may be.

*

BONNIE FORSHEY

Bonnie's son Billy

died in 1993 at age 16

I post a memorial on Billy's birthdate, anniversary date, and all holidays. I will never forget my son. I had him in my life for sixteen years and miss him terribly. I put flowers on his grave, and I cry every time.

*

LAURA HABEDANK

Laura's brother Brian

died in 2010 at age 35

It's been so important to me to not let these days go by unacknowledged. I have a variety of things that I do that help me to get through these days. I do any and all of the following: order pizza and watch Brian's favorite movie, look through pictures of him, watch the photographic memorial DVD my dad put together, light a candle for Brian, listen to some of his favorite music, take a walk to the tree where I've spread some of his ashes or write a letter to him.

I have some wonderful friends who have joined me on some of these occasions and are gracious enough to listen to me share stories about Brian and my favorite memories of him, and offer a shoulder and a box of Kleenex for the times when it's all too much to handle. Those days I definitely experience the loss more profoundly, because it's painful to be celebrating these days without him. But I know I'd feel much worse if I didn't take the time to remember Brian in a way that's special to me and would have been special to him.

*

VICKI HECKROTH
Vicki's son Matthew
died in 2000 at age 17

For Matthew's birthday we usually go away and get together with his sisters and their families for a short vacation. I used to go up and decorate his gravesite, but stopped because too many things were being stolen. I still try to go there to at least visit him on those days. In the beginning, we released balloons for him with messages in them.

*

MARLISE MAGNA
Marlise's fiancé Blaine
died in 2010 at age 36

I tell my close friends and family when his birthday and death anniversaries come up. Usually on his birthday I celebrate his life, but always feel a deep pang of sadness and empathy for his mom, seeing as how Blaine was her only child.

On his birthday I will always think about him, our past, what could have been. It's a day I am always apprehensive about for weeks beforehand, and I tend to stay at home and keep to myself. I always feel such guilt, and the questions pop up more than usual. These last two years it has been bittersweet, as it's also my brother's wedding anniversary. At his wedding, I cried nonstop and people assumed it was due to joy for my brother.

*

MARCELLA MALONE
Marcella's brother Michael
died in 2014 at age 20

Michael's death being only a year and a half ago, my family hasn't really established any traditions for these days. The wound is simply too deep for that. On what would have been his twenty-first birthday, just six months after his passing, we hosted a memorial lantern launch from the high school's old football field, where he did much of his playing and made many great memories. It was nice to be surrounded that day by all the friends and family who loved him. The event was beautiful, despite the wind making it almost impossible to get a lantern in the air. I know Michael got some smiles out of our struggles.

Since then we have not had any special events, nor do we get together. Instead, we have made it a goal within our family and a plea to our Facebook community to complete acts of kindness toward others on these days in Michael's memory. You never know the struggles going on in someone's life. Even something as simple as a smile could improve someone's day or even save his or her life. As I perform these acts, I make sure to leave a note with an encouraging message and some words about that day's significance to me and the amazing person my brother was.

These days also make me remember the importance of family, and I take the time on each of them to make sure they all know how much they are loved, whether it be in person or via the phone. Much of my family does the same. It's truly the little things that make these days pass a little easier.

*

JULIE MJELVE
Julie's husband Cameron
died in 2011 at age 42

Initially, acknowledging the birthday and anniversary of my husband's death was difficult. It was very emotional just to decide what to do. My husband was buried in a different city from where we live, so he could be in the family cemetery. So it's a bit of an outing to get there, and my children are still quite young. But to my surprise, my young children have been my biggest help in figuring it all out, as well as coping with it.

It started on the first anniversary of Cameron's death. I wanted to take them to the gravesite, but I didn't want it to be a terrible, sad day. I wanted to acknowledge his memory and acknowledge our grief, but mourning to me is more about remembering and honoring than it is about negative emotions. So we took flowers to the gravesite. Each child gets their own little flower arrangement so they can individually take part in the mourning ritual rather than just observing it. After we visited the gravesite we went to a lake for the afternoon. The next year, we followed our grave visit with a lovely picnic at the local spray park. The kids initiated that, and we now also go on Father's Day, as well as on my husband's birthday.

My family has been able to approach it with a sense of importance instead of tragedy, and I think that really helps me deal with my emotions on those dates. It has also evolved as to who comes to the grave with us. My husband's parents live in a town nearby, so we have begun picking them up on the way, and making it more of a family event, which also helps to keep us connected, helps us remember that we are all part of my husband's family. We never spend a long time in the cemetery. We put flowers on my husband's grave as well as the graves of other family members in that same cemetery. Then we often go for dinner or dessert with his parents. It has become a nice time of connecting. There is still sadness over his loss, but the importance of remembering stands out overall, and the sadness is more in the background.

*

BRIDGET PARK
Bridget's brother Austin
died in 2008 at age 14

My family and I try to do something my brother liked to do, or eat his favorite food on his birthday, anniversary, etc. However, the anniversary is very difficult to acknowledge, because it is during Thanksgiving, usually one to three days after the holiday. We try to be around family and keep spirits high, because it is really easy to slip into a dark mindset.

My brother's birthday is the hardest for me to celebrate. Every year that goes by and in which he would have grown older, it makes me sad that we are not growing and experiencing life together. I am now twenty years old, and he would be twenty-two if he were still alive. What pains me the most is not having him there with me and not having a life together. I think about how it would have been to send him off to college or see him fall in love and get married. It is all the missed memories and milestones that hurt the most to me. His birthday is also very hard because he and my dad share the same birthday. My dad feels very guilty and sad on this day, because it is just not the same without my brother.

The key for getting through these hard holidays is having loved ones around me and keeping my brother's memory alive. I focus on the beautiful life he lived and not the tragic death he suffered. I think about the memories we were fortunate enough to have together, and I make sure to count them as one of my many blessings in my life.

*

GRACE YOUNG
Grace's son Jack died
in 2007 on his 27th birthday

Since our boy died on his birthday, we have only one anniversary each year. We try to celebrate it the same way we did in his lifetime, with family, cake, balloons, and memories of the good times we shared. We often walk to his grave and light fireworks.

*

It's okay to cry.
Giving in to the tears is terrifying,
like freefalling to earth without a parachute.
But it's vital to our wellbeing as we
process the deep anguish.
LYNDA CHELDELIN FELL

*

CHAPTER SEVEN

THE HOLIDAYS

The only predictable thing about grief is that it's unpredictable. -LYNDA CHELDELIN FELL

The holiday season comes around like clockwork, and for those in mourning, this time of year brings a kaleidoscope of emotions. If the grief is still fresh, the holidays can be downright raw. How do we navigate the invitations, decorations, and festivities with a heart full of sorrow?

*

KAYLA ARNOLD

Kayla's uncle Tim

died in 2001 at age 34

For me, the holiday season isn't as hard as it is for others, mostly because, due to family dynamics, we didn't really celebrate the holidays together. My parents, my sisters and I would do our own thing with Uncle Tim but generally not over the holidays, so my pain isn't linked to the holidays. I know that not everyone has that situation, and for most people the holidays can be crippling! For me though, what I find hard is Uncle Tim not being at things like graduations, concerts, weddings, babies being born, birthdays, etc. For me, the pain comes from his not being here for the big moments that I know he would have been at if he were still here!

And on a personal level, Uncle Tim and I shared a huge passion for University of Michigan football, so for me football season can be hard! I love football season, I love watching them play, but I often find myself wishing Uncle Tim were here to watch it and experience it with me! Last year I went to my first game at the Big House and I know that if he had been here that would have been an experience I would have had with him! So it's the big things and the passions we had together that are harder for me!

*

CHRISTINE BASTONE
Christine's sister Elizabeth
died in 2012 at age 38

That first year, things were different. But otherwise I pass the holiday season pretty close to the way I used to do before my sister died. Now I have one of those pictures with the pretty online frames for all the different holidays. They are printed. And I like to touch them sometimes. This helps me to feel connected to my sister on the holidays. I also have a three-by-five inch picture of Liz in a frame along with a few fake roses that are at my parents' house, which is where I spend most of my holidays. This helps us to feel like she is still here.

That first year during the holidays, all I felt was her absence. So the picture and the flowers were a successful attempt to not feel her absence quite so much. That first Christmas was absolutely excruciating. My biggest problem with Christmas was that it's a season and not just a day. I had learned to deal with one day, but I was dreadfully unprepared for the season, which lasts about a month. The main reason I was so unprepared for Christmas was that I simply ran out of time. I spent so much time figuring out how to handle all the other holidays, especially Thanksgiving, that unfortunately there was no time left to prepare for Christmas.

These days it might be Thanksgiving that is the worst. My sister's Thanksgiving vacation to Florida in 2011 was the last time I saw her alive. Thanksgiving itself is usually okay, but it's the whole weekend after Thanksgiving that is so very, very painful. Over the last three and a half years, holidays have definitely gotten easier. But that doesn't mean they are easy, or that they will be easy any time soon.

*

SHARON EHLERS
Sharon's best friend Joy died in 2009 at age 52
Sharon's former fiancé John died in 2012 at age 59

Holidays are tough since they were Joy's favorite time of year. She loved the holidays. She died in October, so the holidays were already getting started. The first Thanksgiving was hard because it reminded me of the one Thanksgiving we all spent together in Las Vegas. It had been great. It was relaxing and peaceful. Our families all celebrated together. It was one of the best Thanksgivings ever.

Christmas that first year was also very difficult. I was still a mess. I can remember sitting in my living room thinking of Joy while my children baked. At one point my youngest daughter called for me to come into the kitchen. She told me to look at the cake batter she was about to put in the oven. Sure enough, written in the cake batter was the word Joy. I kid you not. It was there and I took a picture to prove it. This affected all of us, and we started to cry. We realized that Joy was there with us that day. It was a magical gift. What was especially hard during Christmas was seeing "Joy" everywhere I looked. Ornaments. Wreaths. Plaques. Songs. Everything seemed to have Joy written on it. The first store I walked into after she died had shopping bags with Joy written all over them. I nearly broke down right then and there. Needless to say I bought a bag.

Those first few years were very difficult because the holidays were one big reminder that Joy was gone. Seeing her name everywhere I went brought me to tears. I avoided places like Michaels craft store just so I didn't have to see her name everywhere. Now I welcome the holidays and seeing her name. It makes me smile to know *Joy* is everywhere. It's the way it should be. I see these reminders as beautiful signs, reminders of her and our friendship. They are reminders that she is always with me.

John's birthday was November 25, which often fell on Thanksgiving. If it wasn't on Thanksgiving, it was always pretty darn close. We often celebrated both occasions together. So after we broke up, Thanksgivings were difficult. After he died, it became even more unbearable. I just wanted to skip right over that day. It became another reminder that John was gone. Thanksgiving was also the last time he had corresponded with me. Why he took the time to send me an email that last Thanksgiving, I'll never know. Maybe he was missing our Thanksgivings together. I know I still did. Bottom line, Thanksgiving will always be tough. I am not sure I will "get over" our times together, and I don't think I should have to. They were a big part of my life and gave me many happy memories that I plan to cherish always.

As for the other holidays, they have been tough but not as difficult as Thanksgiving, Christmas with the children, New Year's Eve toasts, and Valentine's Day dinners. I think I had been grieving those memories since John and I ended our relationship. His death just brought them all to the forefront again. Now I just take them one occasion at a time.

*

BONNIE FORSHEY
Bonnie's son Billy
died in 1993 at age 16

I used to go all out on holidays, but now I don't celebrate. I got rid of all my decorations and don't do anything. I try to block everything out of my mind. I turn off my phone and try to sleep through the holidays. Nothing is the same anymore.

*

LAURA HABEDANK
Laura's brother Brian
died in 2010 at age 35

The only holidays that really sting are Thanksgiving and Christmas, as those were the ones that were the most important to Brian and to our whole family. Brian absolutely adored Thanksgiving, because he loved food and he loved football, both of which he could get a whole bunch of on that day. There was something so soothing about being with family, playing games and laughing, enjoying a large, lovely meal and then falling asleep on the couch to the soothing sound of a football game on the TV.

Christmas is extra hard on me because I have so many fond memories of that time of year. I so adored shopping for presents for Brian; we knew each other so well and always had fun picking out great things for each other and thoroughly enjoyed watching each other open the gifts we exchanged. It often involved at least one gag gift that left us crying tears of laughter. And Brian had just about the best laugh of anyone in the world. It was so incredibly contagious, and I loved being able to bring that out in him so much.

With Brian gone, and all my grandparents gone, I have so little family left that I've pretty much lost most of my interest in the holidays, because the people who made them so special aren't here anymore. I don't get as much enjoyment out of the foods, sounds, sights, and traditions that go along with that time of year anymore. I guess because it's all a reminder of the things I've lost along the way. I have great friends who have welcomed me as part of their family celebrations and I appreciate it so very much but it's hard not to feel out of place there; I find myself looking around the table, at the siblings joking with one another and just aching with jealousy on the inside because I so badly want what they have and I can't have it.

For Christmas and for Brian's birthday I've made it a new tradition to either buy gifts for those less fortunate or donate money to suicide awareness organizations in his memory, because it feels good to give to others when I'm hurting—to turn the pain into something good for someone else.

*

VICKI HECKROTH
Vicki's son Matthew
died in 2000 at age 17

For Thanksgiving and Christmas we adopt families through GLASS in Matthew's memory and the others who are represented. For Thanksgiving, we take turkeys along with all of the fixings to several families. For Christmas we take gifts for children, to people who are less fortunate, using the money we would normally have spent on our loved ones. It gives me a good feeling to know we are doing something that would make our loved ones proud as we bring joy to others. Thanksgiving is the most painful because it is the one holiday when the entire family is always together. That empty chair is always noticeable. Matthew passed away in November, so the pain is always greater that month.

CHAPTER EIGHT

THE BELONGINGS

Of all possessions, a friend is the most precious.
- HERODOTUS

Our loved one's belongings are a direct connection to what once was. Many of us are, at some point, tasked with accepting that the tangible souvenirs from our loved ones are material items that must be dealt with. When does the time come to address the task of sorting out the memory-laden belongings, and how does one begin?

*

KAYLA ARNOLD
Kayla's uncle Tim
died in 2001 at age 34

To handle my uncle's belongings, my parents, my aunt, a few of my uncle's friends, my sisters and myself went over to Uncle Tim's house and packed up the items. My aunt gave multiple things that were his to my sisters and me for us to keep, to remember him with. She kept many things that were his and said that when she was ready she would pass them on. When we were done, the rest of Uncle Tim's stuff was left in the house, because my grandparents ended up moving into the house and living there.

For my sixteenth birthday, my aunt sent me a diamond and ruby necklace that Uncle Tim gave her. She said that she felt he would want me to have it! When I graduated high school she sent me Uncle Tim's class ring, senior necklace, and letterman jacket! These are all items that I cherish and feel blessed to have! Through the years, other items and pictures have been passed down to us as my aunt gets to the point where she feels she can let them go.

*

EMILY BARNHARDT
Emily's friend and roommate Hannah
died in 2014 at age 20

It's common knowledge that after a loss, a loved one's belongings must eventually be taken care of. There are things that have to be addressed and wrapped up, and belongings that must find a new home or be relocated or stored away. It's almost a process that is so obvious and necessary that we sometimes underestimate the impact that the whole experience can have on us.

Losing someone you deeply love is, by itself, an unbearable blow. But also having to handle the very tangible and precious things that were a part of his or her daily life, knowing that those possessions are now your responsibility to decide what to do with, is a trauma in and of itself.

The aftermath of dealing with Hannah's belongings and sorting out the pieces of her life left behind was one of the most traumatic and devastating parts of the process for me. I remember getting that call from Hannah's mom (who lives out of state) early that morning to tell me what had happened. Sometime shortly after we hung up, I remember walking to the open doorway of Hannah's bedroom. I don't know how long I stood there and looked at her room, but the image of her things strewn about as she had left them the day before, will be forever ingrained in my memory. I remember looking at her rumpled bed sheets, her schoolbooks and papers spread across her futon, and her clothes thrown around the room. It seemed inconceivable to me that she would never walk into that room again. This room that depicted Hannah's daily life would never be touched by her again. These things suddenly had no owner, and my mind couldn't fully comprehend that reality.

I didn't expect the process of dealing with Hannah's belongings to have such an impact on me, and I honestly don't think I realized the exact depth of that impact until much later on. It really is its own trauma. Going through her room, I remember being overwhelmed. I knew to set aside the valuables and sentimental things for her family, and I knew they would want some of her clothes. With those aside, I knew I couldn't keep every single thing left of hers, yet getting rid of even a bottle of hairspray felt like I was throwing part of Hannah away. I sorted out the things I knew I wanted to keep myself. But I found that I kept much more than I anticipated. It was just too heartbreaking to part with anything. Every single thing I knew needed to be thrown away or even donated just felt like another part of her I was letting go. It was as if touching the things she touched could connect me to her, almost like fitting your hand inside an old handprint that's indented in dried concrete.

Hannah and I shared the same shoe size and we often borrowed each other's clothes. Her mother said I could keep anything that had significance for me. I will forever be grateful for her parents' generosity and love toward me, and how they have continually honored and valued my relationship with Hannah.

I cherish Hannah's things, that I have them to wear in honor of her. I did feel deeply guilty at the time, however, as I went through her clothes, deciding what items had special memories attached or ones that I'd always loved. It felt wrong, like I was simply going shopping. That wasn't the case at all and, although I knew that, how else can you describe the experience of looking through clothes and having to decide which to keep and which to donate? I also kept other things, like Hannah's favorite makeup. I can't bring myself to use it, so it's tucked away along with other keepsakes, like cards I wrote her that she had kept, or the colleges we made together.

I remember my heart just sank more and more as her room got emptier and emptier in the two months following her death. I donated her furniture to a charity, and when they came for it, I wanted to throw myself on top of it and refuse to let it go. For a few weeks I refused to deal with her belongings altogether. It was heart-wrenching. It became nearly an obsession to keep her room and her things the way they were, for just a little longer. But a little longer was never enough time.

Hannah's daily absence was overwhelming enough as it was. On many days I needed the painful yet comforting feeling of curling up in her bed, smelling her scent and knowing she always slept in that exact spot. I found a comfort in her possessions. I was embarrassed at how often I would just stand and put my hand on something of hers that she often touched or used. It was almost as if touching the things she touched could connect me to her - like placing your hand in an old handprint imbedded in concrete.

Dealing with Hannah's bedroom and her things was a given for me. What I didn't expect, however, was the impact of tying up loose ends in other areas of her life, such as returning her textbooks to our college, dealing with her mail, or the obstacles of closing out bills in her name. Going to pick up Hannah's car from where she had taken her life was especially difficult. Her parents were going to have to sell it so, with the help of a friend, I cleaned out her car so that they wouldn't have to. Hannah always kept an absurd number of things in her car, and cleaning it out brought a flood of countless memories we had together in it. Dealing with the miscellaneous loose ends and pieces made me realize just how much our physical and daily lives were intertwined beyond the realm of friendship and sisterhood.

Each step in the process of dealing with her belongings was another dose of reality, another dose of grief. There was no going back. As more and more of Hannah's things were integrated into my belongings, sent to her family, or donated, that concrete collection of her daily life felt like it was disappearing before my eyes. And I wasn't ready for that. In retrospect, I honestly never would have been ready for that. I never would have been ready to let go of her room being exactly as she left it. It's something no person could ever possibly be ready for and that is, unfortunately, an unbearable process forced upon loved ones after a loss. Some are allowed to, or decide to, wait longer amounts of time before facing this process, while others, like myself, have to face it sooner due to a situation like needing to move.

An outsider might say that I kept too many of Hannah's belongings, and maybe they'd be right. But my personal advice for anyone grieving is to keep anything you even slightly question about wanting. If there's even the slightest resistance to get rid of it, keep it. I've been able to let go of a few of Hannah's things as time has passed. Holding onto the large number of things that I kept is more comforting to me than the opposite situation, where I might have given too much away and wished I could get it back. I hung onto everything I felt the urge to, and I'm thankful that I did.

I've noticed as time has passed that the memories I have with Hannah have become a stronger pathway to feeling connected to her than the connection I feel through her belongings. I will always hang on to special things of hers; they make me feel close to her and are a cherished reminder of the memories we shared. The memories themselves, however, will always be far more valuable than any item that represents them. I'm blessed to be able to have both.

Maybe one day I will be ready to let go of more things, but for now I feel no guilt in keeping anything of Hannah's that I need to.

*

SHARON EHLERS
Sharon's best friend Joy died in 2009 at age 52
Sharon's former fiancé John died in 2012 at age 59

Joy's belongings stayed with her family, but I did ask her husband if I could have a few items. Mostly they were what I had personally given to Joy. A picture of us in a wooden frame that said "Girlfriends," a plaque with a poem about "Best Friends," a guardian angel bracelet I had recently sent to her, a shirt that still smelled of her perfume. It was really all I needed or wanted.

In hindsight, I wished I had asked for a couple more of Joy's belongings, like a piece of her favorite costume jewelry. She was always decked out; it was one of the things that made her Joy. A figurine from the collection of cows in her kitchen - she loved her cow collection, and her kitchen was filled with them. I don't think it would have hurt to have asked for just one.

The last thing I did before I left her house was to sit in her closet one last time. I could tell she had just switched out her summer clothes for her winter ones. Everything was perfectly arranged. But what was more important, everything still smelled like her. I just sat there in her closet and breathed in that smell. I closed my eyes. It was like she was right there with me. I really believe she was.

Once home, I put together a small shrine of the "Girlfriends" photo, the "Best Friends" poem, and a Christmas ornament that says "Joy." It sits above my bed so I can always see it. It's my reminder that she is and was such a beautiful part of my life.

I had quite a few of John's belongings, because we had lived together and been together for so long. Things were either packed away or scattered through the house. Most of the items were actually in the kitchen. John loved kitchen gadgets. He would watch QVC or Home Shopping Network when none of us were home, and buy the craziest kitchen tools, like a grilled cheese flipper where one side was a fork-like thing and the other side was a spatula. After he died, I found myself looking for those things that were "him" and pulling them out. They made me smile. And cry.

We also had furniture together, like my bedroom set and living room set. He also had one of the two reclining chairs I had bought him. Dishes from Thanksgiving. A Christmas tree and ornaments. His bike. Pictures. There were reminders everywhere. It was overwhelming and yet it was also comforting. But those things that were the real vestiges of our relationship were in a single box in the garage. I got that box out within the first few days after John died. I needed to go through it. In it was most of our relationship. I went through each item individually. Dried flowers from special occasions. Cards. Tickets. Receipts. Photographs. Letters. Emails. Clothes. Prayers. Yes, prayers. One of the things I have done over the years is write letters to the angels when I want to "let go" of something and "turn over" the outcome to them. It was a way to help me stop worrying about things I couldn't control. Some people would just not think about those things. That was never me. My brain is always running at warp speed, so I found that if I wrote it down and turned it over to God and the angels, I wouldn't worry about it anymore. So when it came to my relationship with John, it was no different. I would write a letter about something that was difficult or needed healing in our relationship. Once the letter was written, I would file it away and forget about it. I obviously really forgot about them, because I found hundreds of letters I had written. Enough to become a book. I pulled them out and started to read them. "Please help John…" "Please heal John…", and on and on. I was moved to tears. I took a few of them with me up to my bedroom and read them out loud. I did this hoping that John would hear them. Hoping that he would finally understand how much I had loved him. How difficult it had been to let go of our relationship when I really still loved him. How difficult it was to know he was no longer here.

*

BONNIE FORSHEY
Bonnie's son Billy
died in 1993 at age 16

My son was a very loving and giving young man. He was always giving things away to those who less fortunate. He would pick out shoes and clothes, assure me that they fit, and then a couple of days later he would tell me they didn't fit. He was actually buying them for one of his friends whose mother couldn't work. I never got mad; Billy was just so kind and wanted him to have clothes for school, and not be ashamed.

My son had ended his life shortly after school began. His closet was packed with new school clothes and shoes; the tags were still on them. It didn't take me long, because I knew what Billy would have wanted me to do. I called his friend and asked him to come to my house. They were like brothers, and it was so difficult for him to walk in the door. I had brought everything out of Billy's room, and I told him that Billy would want him to have the clothes. They were the same size and everything fit him. He started to cry, and I told him again that Billy would want him to have them. We loaded everything into my car and took them to his house. It was nice to see how proud he was when he wore those clothes. It made me happy.

There was another very poor family down the street. I found out that the youngest child didn't have a bed. I called the father and asked him to come to my house. We disassembled Billy's waterbed and I gave him the entire bedroom set for his son. I also let him take down the basketball hoop, etc., to take home for his son. There was no reason to hold on. Billy would not be returning home, and he would want someone else to have his belongings. That's the kind of unselfish child he was. I miss him so much, but I did what I thought was best.

*

LAURA HABEDANK
Laura's brother Brian
died in 2010 at age 35

Just three days after getting the phone call telling me my only brother had taken his own life, I found myself in his condo with my family cleaning out all his belongings. It felt so wrong being there going through everything he owned; it felt like a betrayal of his privacy in a way. I still hadn't fully grasped that it was real and I fully expected to see him come walking through the door and ask us to knock it off.

It turns out that in his final few months Brian had fallen behind in his mortgage payments because he'd been out of full-time work for a year. That was so unlike him, because he was undoubtedly the most responsible person I'd ever known; the last we spoke about it he had been months ahead in the payments and had money in savings and was doing just fine. But the more depressed he grew, the less drive he had to go out and pursue a job when, in his mind, he wouldn't be around for much longer. The real estate market had taken a terrible turn and the housing values in his neighborhood had dramatically plummeted, and the balance of the loan was far greater than the value of the home. So there we were hastily trying to empty his home of everything he owned as quickly as possible. Some went into the dumpster, some we donated to a neighbor of Brian's who was in need of some furnishings, but the majority of it went into our vehicles and trailer. We planned on getting as much as we could out of there that day, in one trip, and walk away from it. It was all very rushed. I can't adequately explain everything I was feeling that day, but I did feel a bit of shame; we walked away knowing full well that the bank would soon be coming to foreclose on the house. I was embarrassed for Brian, because as responsible as he was, I know he wouldn't have wanted to be remembered for skirting any responsibility, financial or otherwise.

I didn't pay much attention to Brian's things until they were all I had left of him. But after he died, I found myself irrationally attached to anything that belonged to him, anything he had touched. I immediately regretted that we had thrown away anything at all... I suddenly wanted to keep every single pen with which he ever wrote, every sample of his handwriting, every shirt he had ever worn, and every glass from which he had sipped too much vodka throughout the days leading up to his death. They were all precious to me; if he had touched it, I wanted to save it.

We sold his car a few weeks later, and that too felt wrong. I was still holding out hope that it was all just a terrible misunderstanding and he'd show up any day looking for all his stuff. I kept his big TV, and I treasure it so much. I'm sure it sounds silly, but the TV was on when he was found, so I know it was one of the last few things he looked at; it was in the room with him when he died. I have his laptop, and never imagined that someday I'd be typing these horrifying words on it.

There are a few things of Brian's that hold extra-special meaning for me, the things that were extra-special to him. I often wear his Jack Del Rio jersey, his favorite flannel pajama pants, and his favorite hooded sweatshirt. I sleep every night with the blanket I crocheted as a gift for his very last birthday; it was purple and gold for the Minnesota Vikings and he was so proud of it. The police report said Brian had the blanket on his lap when he died. I like to imagine that he felt some comfort having that blanket with him and that he felt as much love for him coming out of that blanket as I put into every single stitch of it.

As much as I value all these things, I'd give anything to be able to trade them all back for just one more day with him.

*

VICKI HECKROTH
Vicki's son Matthew
died in 2000 at age 17

I was cheated out of taking care of Matt's belongings. The day I went back to work, my father came over while we were gone and tore Matt's room apart, getting rid of all of his belongs, ripping the carpet up, tearing down his bed, etc. He then proceeded to tell me that Matt's death was all my fault. That is something I can never get over. I didn't get to keep anything except Matt's wallet and Social Security card. The police took his driver's license. I also have his birth and death certificates. Not nearly enough to remember my son by.

*

MARLISE MAGNA
Marlise's fiancé Blaine
died in 2010 at age 36

I had nothing to do with packing up Blaine's belongings. In fact, sadly I have nothing of his whatsoever aside from a ring I gave him and necklaces of mine that he wore. I currently wear the chain around my neck with a cross pendant. His mom and close family friends almost immediately packed up his belongings. His mom had his computer hacked, and all of Blaine's social media and email accounts were deleted along with our online music pages that contained our published songs. I felt anger at first - but now I realize that to them it probably would have been a constant reminder of what happened.

*

MARCELLA MALONE
Marcella's brother Michael
died in 2014 at age 20

Within the first couple of weeks after Michael's death, the immediate family chose the items they wanted for comfort or remembering him. Other than that, Michael's room and belongings remained sat they were for a couple of months. Entering it was too painful for any of us. About three months later, my cousin came and spent the weekend with my mom to help her start going through Michael's room. They accomplished quite a bit, but mostly just organizing and getting rid of garbage; his room was never very clean. Having neutral support was very helpful and necessary for my mom throughout that task.

Since then, very little has been done. Occasionally someone will go in and look around, but that's about it. Once the one year anniversary had passed, our family began to use his things we needed. I have some of his electronics, and my older brother has Michael's hunting gear. We decided it was better to use it and honor him than let it sit. My parents also gave some of Michael's belongings, like his weight equipment, to his close friends who could use it.

It will be a long time before his room is altered to become something other than his room. Eighteen months just isn't enough to make it seem real that Michael really isn't coming home.

For Christmas this year I am working on a project for my son and nephew with some of Michael's old clothes. Although he never got to meet them, he was excited to be an uncle and I know he's with them. I want to make sure they know him.

*

JULIE MJELVE
Julie's husband Cameron
died in 2011 at age 42

I packed my loved one's stuff primarily by myself, but there were a few instances where friends came to help me. It was a difficult job, and there were things I wish I had done differently.

Everyone has his own opinion about what to keep and what not to keep. There were items that friends encouraged me to give away that I wish I had kept. On the flip side, there were other items that friends encouraged me to keep that I now look back on and think "What in the world did I keep that for?" So it is a difficult task, but I think it's better to keep too much than not enough. You can always go back later and give things away, but you can't get them back once they're gone. It did bring a lot of emotions. I think it's very important to have the right people help you. People who can be understanding and patient with the emotions you are experiencing, and the difficulty you will have giving away an object that seems absolutely mundane and ridiculous to keep in their eyes, but holds incredible memories for you. I cried a lot while I packed my husband's things. It felt as though I was packing away not just his things, but my dreams of our life together. It wasn't just packing random physical items, it was packing away everything I'd hoped for since childhood.

Even now, four years later, I find it very difficult to go through Cameron's things. Some things are easy to give away at this point, and some will even bring a smile to my face as I remember the events they are associated with, which is something I definitely did not experience in the original packing! Some things still bring tears to my eyes as I relive the pain of his loss, and the pain of my lost dreams and goals for our life together. But I find that allowing myself to experience the pain all over again has its healing moments. I have to be careful about how much I do at one time; it can still overwhelm me. But, in small pieces, I also continue to heal.

*

BRIDGET PARK
Bridget's brother Austin
died in 2008 at age 14

My family and I waited a long time to box up my brother's belongings, around six to eight months. We left his room untouched, exactly how he left it, so we could go in there and feel like he was still living in it. I know that my mom would go and sit on Austin's bed and talk to him like she used to when he was alive. It was nice to see all of his stuff and not look deeper than surface level at his belongings and his life. Soon we realized that we needed to move on, and learn how to keep his memory alive in other ways.

*

GRACE YOUNG
Grace's son Jack died
in 2007 on his 27th birthday

Jack lived in Pittsburgh. My husband and son Ben had to make a fourteen-hour drive to pack up Jack's belongings and get his van. Jack lived on the ground floor of a large apartment building. When we first walked in, we could not envision how he could have hanged himself in this tiny apartment with low ceilings. We finally saw the folding chair in the hallway, the cut electrical cord of his vacuum, and the missing screws from the overhead light in the hall by the folding chair. I will never forgive the makers of the movie *Shawshank Redemption* for showing everyone how to kick the chair away. We searched around for a note, but found none. Jack had so many pieces of art, and so many notebooks of poems and drawings. One of the notebooks had a page that said "HI MOM." We solemnly packed up Jack's van with all his things. We asked the neighbors who came out to walk their dogs if they knew Jack, but they just walked away without speaking to us. We headed back home during a large storm. Our town was littered with tree limbs, and the power was out. We reverently carried Jack's things back into his room by candlelight. It was very surreal, and horribly painful.

*

We need to change the culture of this topic and make it okay to speak about mental health and suicide.
LUKE RICHARDSON

*

CHAPTER NINE

THE DARKNESS

Walking with a friend in the dark is better than walking alone in the light. -HELEN KELLER

Suicidal thoughts occur for many in the immediate aftermath of profound loss, yet few readily admit it for fear of being judged or condemned. While there would be no rainbow without the rain, where do we find the energy to fight the storm?

*

KAYLA ARNOLD
Kayla's uncle Tim
died in 2001 at age 34

I have in no way ever had suicidal thoughts since losing my uncle! The pain, suffering, and agony that I and my family have had to go through for the last fourteen years is pain and emotions I would NEVER wish upon anyone, let alone put my family through it again! I did get depressed after losing my uncle, as did most of my family. But suicide was never a thought. I can't even imagine putting my family and friends through that! After experiencing being left behind by a family member who chose to take his life and leave me willingly, I would never do that to my loved ones.

I have used my own personal experience with suicide, and the pain and suffering that those left behind feel, to help others. And I have helped stop a few friends who were suicidal by showing them they had someone to talk to, and talking to them about my experience and the pain I have been through.

*

EMILY BARNHARDT
Emily's friend and roommate Hannah
died in 2014 at age 20

When I look back on the deepest valley of my grief, all the memories and events of that time period are clouded by this looming dark shadow. Even in remembering routine tasks or random events I attended, there's a darkness present in those memories. It's almost as if I see the color black in correlation with any memory from that time period.

It makes sense to me though, because nothing has ever felt more haunting and dark than losing someone I dearly loved to suicide. Nothing is more haunting than those images I picture in my mind of how she died, all the unanswered questions, the sorrow I feel over the amount of pain Hannah was in, and the torturous hell I've put myself through in trying to understand.

The color black is pretty much associated with darkness. In a closed room with no light, that black void is all one can see. And suicide occurs when a person sees just that—a blinding dark void consuming the space where light, life, and hope are supposed to be.

Suicidality is a blinding darkness that overtakes the soul, obscuring one's view of reality, canceling out rationality and casting all hopeful facets of one's life into a seemingly dismal and black abyss. After her death, suicide was honestly all I thought about; not in terms of feeling suicidal myself, but due to suddenly being thrown into a world of grief because of it. For a long time,

124

whenever I would think of Hannah (which felt like constantly), the overall darkness of the concept of suicide would also come to mind.

I believe there are two separate griefs in the loss of a loved one by suicide. There is the overall grief over their death, and then there is the grief over the fact that they died by suicide. Suicide grief brings a complex myriad uniquely horrific emotions, thoughts and questions. Grief alone feels dark enough, and death by suicide can multiply that darkness immensely.

It was an emotional rollercoaster for me, and still is at times. But it's become a little more bearable and gentler now than it used to be. In the first year of grief, there were a few frightening and painful nights where the despair felt consuming and the tears felt lethal. I wanted to find hope in knowing that life goes on. But the thought of life moving forward made me incredibly sad, because I ached to go back. On those nights, I felt like Hannah's pain had transferred to me, like catching a virus. In my desperate striving to understand why and find the answers, it was as if I unintentionally picked up the heavy burden and pain that she had been carrying. The anguish and despair Hannah felt that night became my own in a way, and it terrified me. I couldn't escape it; the constant exposure to the subject of suicide and the weight that it carries weighed heavily on me.

It was during those few nights when the grief felt so consuming and dark, that I wondered if I would ever feel okay again. The threat of hopelessness and the depth of grief took me to a dark place, where the possibility of suicide did flicker across my mind, honestly. I knew I would never allow that to be an option, and while I couldn't control the fact that the thought crossed my mind, I knew that I could control what I chose to do with it and how I handled it. I reminded myself that negative thoughts rarely depict the truth of a situation. I was deeply ashamed that the possibility of suicide even crossed my mind, even though I knew I didn't choose or ask for it to. I found out that it is actually common in people who lose someone to suicide to have moments where they might feel that way themselves. Research shows that people who lose someone to suicide are at a higher risk to feel that way as well, so it's extremely important for grievers to take care of themselves, give themselves compassion, and reach out for support when they need it. Knowing that it is common actually gave me the assurance that I wasn't alone in it or crazy and that it didn't mean I was failing; it was an effect of my grief and not my own personal reality.

I was afraid to reach out to anyone in those dark moments though, because of my shame and fear that their reaction might only make me feel worse. So in those moments I reminded myself that the grief and devastation couldn't kill me, though the crushing pain of it certainly felt capable at times. And I knew that if the pain itself couldn't kill me, that meant there is hope. I wasn't doomed. I reminded myself of my loved ones, and how I could never bear causing them the grief and devastation I currently felt from Hannah's death.

I reminded myself of my faith. I believe God has a plan for my life, and I don't want to miss out on it. I know He created me for a purpose, and I want to fulfill that purpose. I believe there is no amount of pain He cannot carry me through, no amount of trauma He cannot heal, and no amount of loss so great that He cannot give me a feeling of restoration in my life again.

On those painful nights, I reminded myself that my story isn't over. I didn't want it to be. I wanted to see God's promises fulfilled in my life. I wanted to glorify Him. I knew He would find a way to bring something beautiful from my grief, and I wanted to be able to witness it. And I already have! God opened a random and unexpected door that connected me to Lynda, the author of this book series. And I feel so honored and blessed to be a part of this, to share my words and my heart with the hope that something I say will touch another's heart, make someone feel less alone, validate someone in his or her struggle, or give someone the hope and encouragement to carry on. Being able to do something good out of what I've gone through, that can help or encourage others, is what keeps me going on the hard and difficult days.

*

CHRISTINE BASTONE
Christine's sister Elizabeth
died in 2012 at age 38

I have had suicidal thoughts since Liz died. Although that very first night after I learned that she had died, and I learned how it feels to lose a loved one this way, I decided that I would never so much as consider suicide ever again. But unfortunately life doesn't work that way. I would soon have such thoughts. They come on very suddenly. They also come on very strong, but thankfully they last usually only a few minutes. The longest they last is a few hours.

They were really scary at first. I would go to bed and just lie there, not moving, until the feeling went away. I felt that if I didn't let myself do anything, I couldn't hurt myself. Even though they were so short-lived, I still wanted to find a different way to deal with them. So I found two friends who, I could share with when I felt that way. A lot of times what I shared with them was just something I needed to say. It wasn't even necessarily what I believed, it was just the thoughts going around and around in my head. And getting them out of my head seemed to help.

I also read a few things that helped me. The first thing was that suicide happens when a person's pain exceeds his or her resources to handle that pain. And while that is simple, and being suicidal is complex, I do not find it simplistic. More than once I have taken a piece of paper, put a line down the middle of it, and written "Reduce Pain" on one side and "Increase Resources" on the other, and then listed ways that I could do both. Doing that exercise, even before any changes are actually made, has helped all by itself.

The second thing was that when you're suicidal, you have a need to change something for which you would rather die than go on living without. And to use suicidal feelings as a catalyst for that change, it makes the feelings empowering instead of so negative. I love this. And this is how I try to look at any suicidal feelings now.

So, yes, I have had thoughts of suicide since Liz's death. But, thankfully, they have been just thoughts, and I have not been actively suicidal. And thankfully I have also found constructive ways to deal with them.

*

SHARON EHLERS
Sharon's best friend Joy died in 2009 at age 52
Sharon's former fiancé John died in 2012 at age 59

This will be my shortest response. No, I have not thought about suicide since Joy and John died. I have been sadder than I ever thought I could imagine. I have said that it felt like my heart and my soul had been ripped out of my body after they died. But I have never felt like taking my own life. I have seen firsthand what it does to the people left behind, and I love my children and family too much to do that to them.

I made sure that I practiced self-care when I was grieving. Eating as best as I could (when I felt like it). Trying to rest. Using the Japanese art form Reiki to keep me relaxed and less stressed out, even if it was only for a few hours here and there. But I really think what kept me going through the grief was the signs I received after Joy and John both died. The signs made it seem less final. Less ominous. Less finite. I knew they were around. I knew they were okay. I knew they were finally at peace. In turn, they knew they were loved.

Joy sent me butterflies, songs, the smell of her perfume, and "Joy" written in the cake batter (red velvet, by the way) to name a few. John sent me a pelican that would always be there when I walked at the beach, "our" songs on the radio, and especially dreams. The dreams have never stopped. In fact, there are days when I still wake up feeling like they had actually happened. It's in those moments that I know they are both always with me and never too far away. It's those things that made getting through my grief much more bearable.

*

BONNIE FORSHEY
Bonnie's son Billy
died in 1993 at age 16

Yes, I thought about suicide a lot. I even attempted suicide, but always failed. I finally went on antidepressants and am able to cope. I have a daughter and two grandsons now. I have to stick around for them. I think my attempts failed because my work on earth is not complete.

*

LAURA HABEDANK
Laura's brother Brian
died in 2010 at age 35

Because of my own lifelong struggle with depression, I've thought about ending my own life more times than I could possibly count. But the level of despair and worthlessness I felt following Brian's death was immeasurable. I had lost all hope and couldn't possibly imagine myself having any quality of life at all if I even managed to survive. I couldn't shake the feeling of resenting him for taking his life when that was what I had wanted for myself so many times. Now that he had gone and done that, it would make me a real asshole to do that and leave Mom and Dad with no children at all. I hated the agony I was experiencing and wanted so badly to die. But there was nothing I could do about it; I felt as though he had stolen that option from me, and that upset me.

That being said, I've never been angry at him for his choice, because I've spent so much time in that place myself. I know how it feels to be experiencing a sadness of such depth and intensity and for such long periods of time that you aren't even capable of seeing any way through it at all. I know exactly what it's like to go to bed at night in such emotional agony that your body actually hurts and you pray so hard that you just don't wake up in the morning, because you've run out of strength to pretend anymore. I know this wasn't a decision that Brian took lightly and he fought longer and harder than he really had any energy for simply because I asked him to. So even now, after five years, I still have yet to experience the "anger" stage of the grief cycle, and I honestly don't foresee it ever happening. I have felt only compassion for him, because I've felt that despair and wouldn't wish it on anyone, and I certainly wouldn't blame someone for making that choice for him or herself in the end. In fact, I've found myself feeling painfully envious of him for seeking that peace, because I've had so much difficulty finding any of it myself.

I've been writing letters to Brian to express my feelings, and it helps me feel as though I'm talking directly to him and helps me process my thoughts a little more clearly. But every now and then I still fall back on my old habit of self-injury when I'm too overwhelmed to even begin to collect my thoughts and am desperate for a quick release. To anyone who doesn't understand, I'm sure it seems a barbaric ritual (and possibly counterintuitive) to cause oneself physical harm as a means to feel better, but I wouldn't do it if it didn't work. It happens so rarely now but every now and then all the sadness becomes too much to handle and I resort to the ironic "comfort" of the razor blade. It's certainly not ideal, but it helps and for now that's enough for me.

*

VICKI HECKROTH
Vicki's son Matthew
died in 2000 at age 17

Yes, several times. However, since Matthew's death I started a suicide prevention and awareness group in his honor. So when I feel that way, I always get immediate help. I feel I would be letting so many people down by committing suicide when I preach to them that suicide is never the answer. Plus I know how much it will hurt my family again. I could never put them through that.

*

MARLISE MAGNA
Marlise's fiancé Blaine
died in 2010 at age 36

I have been admitted to the hospital and ended on life support quite a few times after Blaine's passing. At one stage the emergency room knew me on a first-name basis, I was there so often.

I am a very open person, so I wear my heart on my sleeve, and people did suspect I would attempt suicide. Eventually, after prolonged intensive psychotherapy, I realized it just wasn't my time and not fair on the people getting left behind. A friend asked me one day whether I want to be remembered as "the girl who killed herself" or would I rather leave a legacy. After that I never tried again. I still have deep sorrow and despair, but I also have faith and that keeps me going.

*

MARCELLA MALONE
Marcella's brother Michael
died in 2014 at age 20

In the super-emotional state after losing my brother/best friend so suddenly and beginning my third trimester with my first child, yes, I had a few suicidal thoughts. The pain seemed too harsh some moments, and it led to wondering if it would be easier to join Michael, if it would be easier to end my life rather than leave others to deal with the burden of my grief. The thoughts were not very calculated and rarely lasted more than a couple of hours, but they happened. Consciously I know I couldn't do it, though. I have too much to live for. Just looking into my sons eyes, I know the devastating impact of such a decision.

*

JULIE MJELVE
Julie's husband Cameron
died in 2011 at age 42

I have had thoughts of suicide since my spouse passed away. My life has been very difficult; I'm raising three very young children alone. At the time of my husband's passing, my children were three-and-a-half years-old, two years-old, and five months-old. My youngest daughter has Down syndrome, and it has been difficult at times coping with the extent of her disability and all the appointments. Furthermore, my oldest child who is now eight, was diagnosed with Tourette's syndrome six months ago, adding to the our household challenges. Three months ago, my middle child who is now six, was diagnosed with an anxiety disorder. This has all been a lot to handle, especially without a spouse to talk to, debrief with, and make decisions together. There have been many, many appointments and therapies and, as a result, I am not working which creates an extra financial strain. My family does not live in the same city as I do, except for my dad who is here only for a few months of the year. So, family support is minimal at best.

So, yes; thoughts of suicide do occur to me when I'm overwhelmed. Fortunately though, I am able to focus on my children and how much they need me. What would happen to them if I too were gone? It is a strong motivator for me to continue moving forward.

Also, I have learned how to pray. I used to pray for God to take away the difficult situations, and struggled to understand why he did not lighten my load so it was not quite so overwhelming. But, over time, I learned to take a different focus. Now I pray for God to give me strength to deal with the situations that arise. I pray for God to provide through finances as well as people who can help support me. And now he answers. Well, he answered before too, he just said "no." The answers may not come in ways I expected or preferred, especially the timelines. But if I pay attention, the strength to survive another day comes, and he provides. We have a roof over our head, food on our table, and new friends who help us through the tough times.

*

GRACE YOUNG
Grace's son Jack died
in 2007 on his 27th birthday

I have not had any thoughts of suicide since my son died, because I had to be strong for the rest of my family. My mom was devastated by Jack's death. Since she has multiple health issues, and I am her caregiver, I had to help her through her grief as well as my own.

*

133

I walked a mile with Pleasure;
She chatted all the way.
But left me none the wiser
for all she had to say.

I walked a mile with Sorrow;
And ne'er a word said she.
But, oh! The things I
learned from her,
when Sorrow walked with me.
ROBERT BROWNING HAMILTON

*

CHAPTER TEN

THE FRIENDS

Remember, you don't need a certain number of friends, just a number of friends you can be certain of. -UNKNOWN

When we are mourning, some of our friendships undergo transitions. Some bonds remain steady, dependable and faithful. Some we sever by choice. And, perhaps unexpectedly, new friends enter our life, bringing renewed hope rich with possibilities. But what about your loved one's friends? Do you keep in touch with them?

*

KAYLA ARNOLD
Kayla's uncle Tim
died in 2001 at age 34

I have had interaction with some of my uncle's friends, not a lot, but here and there throughout the last fourteen years. I enjoy it, because they were important to my uncle and that makes them important to me. They have gone through the same emotions, feelings and pain that my family and I did. Therefore we have an understanding of the pain of missing my uncle.

So I find comfort in seeing people who loved and cared for my uncle as much as I did and still do. It is also always fun to see reactions from them, because I don't see them a lot. I was twelve when my uncle passed away and now I am twenty-six, so a lot has changed. But it is still comforting to see people who loved him.

*

EMILY BARNHARDT
Emily's friend and roommate Hannah
died in 2014 at age 20

From the opposite perspective, as a friend of Hannah's, I have really appreciated staying in touch with her family. Not only have we stayed in touch, but I've grown closer to her mother and have met more members of Hannah's family, like her grandparents, her aunt, and her cousin when I flew out to Tennessee to visit them. Each of Hannah's family members have touched my heart. They truly are a beautiful family and they feel like family to me now. I've been blessed to get to know them better since Hannah passed. I've cherished my times with them (whether in person or on the phone), not only because I see or hear parts of Hannah in all of them, but also because they are just an incredibly sweet, warm, and loving family. There's no question where Hannah got those wonderful traits from. I can't begin to imagine their pain, but their love and support for me amid their own grief means the world to me. I truly feel honored to know them.

Family came up often in my conversations with Hannah. We talked about how grateful we were for our families, and we counted our blessings. Hannah loved her family dearly. Her heart lit up as she spoke of memories or hearing their voices on the phone. Hannah's family brought her joy and life and unconditional love. And after getting to know them more myself, I can totally see why. Hannah once told me that her family was her greatest blessing, and I believe it.

*

CHRISTINE BASTONE
Christine's sister Elizabeth
died in 2012 at age 38

Sadly I do not really know any of Liz's friends. I did receive a condolence message from one of her previous neighbors. But, because I didn't know the guy, Facebook put it in my "other" folder and I didn't see it for months. I was so upset for a while that such an important message did not go to my inbox. I also very briefly connected with two people that Liz went to school with. The only other thing I did in the hopes of connecting with a few of her friends was to write a comment on Liz's MySpace profile saying that she had died. But nobody responded. Although to be fair, they probably didn't see it. I would absolutely love to connect with some of Liz's friends! It would be so cool to connect with someone who knew her in a slightly different way than I did. And I am sad that so far, at least, I have not been able to do so.

*

SHARON EHLERS
Sharon's best friend Joy died in 2009 at age 52
Sharon's former fiancé John died in 2012 at age 59

Since Joy and I had worked together for years, many of our mutual coworkers are still a part of my life. What's interesting, though, is that none of them ever bring up Joy's name or what happened to her. Usually I am the one to do it. I do it for a few reasons. One, not everyone knows how to handle Joy's suicide, and if I bring it up I am showing them it is okay to talk about it. Two, I bring it up to make sure they remember the wonderful person Joy was to all of us. She was a good person and deserves to be remembered. As for Joy's circle of friends in Las Vegas, I don't have any contact with them or, sadly, with her husband. At some point after Joy's death I became angry with him. He said he was going to have us out to help spread Joy's ashes at Lake Mead near Las Vegas, but he never called. I also couldn't understand what had happened on the day Joy died. What transpired between our talk and Joy's decision to take her own life? What had been said? I didn't think her husband was being honest with me, so I pulled away. I honestly couldn't deal with it. Over time, I eventually reached out to him when I heard his mother and stepfather had passed away, but I haven't gone beyond that. I know that someday I will talk with him, but I am just not ready yet.

As with Joy, many of my mutual friends with John are still part of my life. Again like with Joy, none of them ever bring up his name or what happened to him. I am the one to do it for the reasons stated above. As for John's friends, the interaction went away after John and I ended our relationship.

In hindsight, if I had been thinking straight after his death, I probably would have reached out to some of John's friends. It just didn't feel right at the time. My head was too clouded with my own grief and sadness. I do, however, keep in regular contact with John's mom. After his death it was heartbreaking to talk with her. She didn't understand why he had killed himself. I couldn't shed much insight into that other than to say he had changed over the years. She agreed. She had also found out that John had left no will and no money. There were bills that still had to be paid. It made me angry that his two children, who were only in their early twenties, and his elderly mother were left with such a mess.

About two years after his death, John's mom fell and ended up in the hospital, where she stayed for almost a year. There was no one in the local Virginia area to help her. John's children were off in other states at graduate school. I called her as much as I could. Again, I became angry that John's suicide had left her alone. I was angry that John was so caught up in himself that he couldn't even make sure he provided for his mother and children. I can see why they say people who commit suicide are selfish. In John's case, I feel very much that way. Maybe that anger will go away one day. Mostly it just makes me sad; it just breaks my heart.

*

BONNIE FORSHEY

Bonnie's son Billy

died in 1993 at age 16

I still talk to Billy's friends and even his girlfriend. We have stayed in touch, and they email or message me every year on certain days. It's nice to know that they have not forgotten me and that they loved my son enough to stay in contact with me.

*

LAURA HABEDANK

Laura's brother Brian

died in 2010 at age 35

I live so far away from home now that I never see anyone who knew Brian except for during my rare visits home to Minnesota. If I'm being honest, I haven't been back home as often as I probably should, because I'm bombarded with memories when I'm there. It's not as though I have my head buried in the sand about it or anything, because it's still on my mind every day. But I guess those thoughts are a little less overwhelming when I'm not also surrounded by all the places we spent time together and all the people who knew Brian. It's been easier for me to have some distance from all of that and have my very own life here in Texas.

Growing up, our house was where Brian and his best friends hung out nearly all the time, so I basically had a whole extra set of surrogate brothers while I was growing up. It's been hard for me seeing them go through all the amazing changes in adulthood that

I haven't had the opportunity to experience with my own brother: getting married, having children and building their dream homes. I'm so happy for them, but there is a part of me that aches because I never got the chance to see these milestones realized for Brian, too. I will admit there have been moments when I've felt that my attachment to his closest friends has become unhealthy; I miss my brother so much, and they are the closest thing to a brother I have left now. I feel protective of them, but I also feel painfully needy and inferior for reaching out to them like I do at times.

This misplaced attachment is not exactly a new phenomenon for me. The first significant death in my life was that of my grandpa, my mom's father, during my senior year in high school. I loved him so much, and was just devastated when he died. At his funeral I became very fixated on his brother, Harold, who was the spitting image of my grandpa. I knew it wasn't him, but Harold looked so much like him that I just stayed glued to his side that day because he was now the closest thing I had left to the real thing.

Last month I went home to Minnesota for a visit after not having been there in over two years. I had the chance to see a few of Brian's closest friends, and it meant the world to me to spend time with them and talk about him. To be able to share memories about Brian and know that others miss him too is so precious to me.

*

VICKI HECKROTH
Vicki's son Matthew
died in 2000 at age 17

I have had interaction only with Matthew's girlfriend and his best friend. Seeing them moving on with families of their own hurts me immensely. It always makes me wonder what Matt's life would be like at this time. Would he be married? Would he have kids of his own? Would he have gone to college? What would his career be? It is like rubbing salt into a raw wound. Yet at the same time Matt's best friend allows me to be a part of his kids' lives, which is a blessing. So it is sort of a win-lose situation for me.

*

MARLISE MAGNA

Marlise's fiancé Blaine

died in 2010 at age 36

My circle of friends has slowly but surely changed since his passing. The friends who have stayed behind still treat me the same. I think the fact that I've always been open about my feelings has helped them understand and not feel they need to wear kid gloves around me.

*

MARCELLA MALONE

Marcella's brother Michael

died in 2014 at age 20

Since Michael's passing, interactions with his friends are very comforting for me. Talking to the people who saw him most during his final couple of years helped me to get to know him better and remember the amazing person he was. Growing up, I became sort of a surrogate big sister to many of Michael's friends. I began to truly care for them and their role in his life. Honestly, I can't imagine not seeing them anymore. It would be like a larger chunk of my life was gone. They help me to remember Michael and manage my grief. While there are a couple of exceptions to this, I love watching them grow. I love being part of their continued existence, despite the sadness it brings me that I will never get to see Michael accomplish the same goals they have.

141

*

JULIE MJELVE
Julie's husband Cameron
died in 2011 at age 42

The interactions with my husband's friends have decreased significantly. However, I have maintained an excellent relationship with his parents. I was surprised by this originally. I wasn't sure how they would want to interact with me. After all, their son, the reason they know me, is now gone. However, they have embraced me fully and have striven to ensure that I and my children are taken care of. They have completely taken on the role of grandparents. We even pick them up and visit the gravesite together. Our bond continues to increase, probably more so than if my husband had still been alive.

*

BRIDGET PARK
Bridget's brother Austin
died in 2008 at age 14

My brother's friends and I are now becoming more like friends than acquaintances, because when my brother died I was thirteen and they were all sixteen, so there was quite an age gap. But now that I am older, it is easier to befriend them. We talk about memories of my brother and how we all miss him. It was nice to hear all their stories and memories, because I can imagine my brother doing these things with them and laughing at these jokes that they are now telling me. It makes me happy to see how loved and missed my brother is, and that he did not leave this earth unnoticed or unloved, but he left this earth along with so many people who cherish him.

*

GRACE YOUNG
Grace's son Jack died
in 2007 on his 27th birthday

I am so thankful for Jack's friends. They are the ones who came up with the idea for our annual music benefit, Particle Accelerator, in memory of Jack Young Jr. They did not see the signs of Jack's depression, and wanted to do something to help others see the signs and hopefully prevent more deaths. They keep us in their lives, call and stop by often, and are so supportive and kind.

*

Even the smallest star shines in darkness
-FINISH PROVERB

*

CHAPTER ELEVEN

THE RELATIONSHIPS

I have found the paradox that if you love until it hurts, there can be no more hurt, only more love.
-MOTHER TERESA

For many of us, familial relationships are the cornerstones that help us stay sane; they keep us laughing, learning, and loving. We speak one another's language and often finish one another's sentences. Sometimes, however, loss touches us in different ways. What family relations, if any, were impacted by your loss?

*

KAYLA ARNOLD
Kayla's uncle Tim
died in 2001 at age 34

I would have to say that for the most part my relationships were not impacted in a bad way. My family already had a lot of family dynamics going on that made my relationship with a few of my family members an already distant relationship. But I can certainly say that one relationship that was never the same, and will never be the same since my uncle passed, is my relationship with my grandma. I can't say I always had the best relationship with her in the first place, but after my uncle died she did and said

145

somethings that even to this day I remember! I was only twelve, and those comments stuck in my head! My uncle and my grandpa were the glue that held that side of my family together, and my uncle passed on May 3, 2001, and my grandpa died from lung cancer May 5, 2002. When they passed it seemed like my grandma felt she didn't have to try anymore. Our relationship declined more and more over the years.

Many different events happened that continued to place more distance between us, and now we do not talk and haven't seen each other or spoken in years. It is sad, but in all honesty it is her loss. Even though my relationship with my grandma was further damaged after the deaths of my loved ones, thankfully my uncle's death did bring my immediate family (my parents, my sisters and myself) closer together. We all suffered and grieved in our own ways, but it brought us together and made us a close-knit family. So out of the negative there was some positive.

Overall, my relationships were not affected, but there were some setbacks and some improvements!

*

EMILY BARNHARDT
Emily's friend and roommate Hannah
died in 2014 at age 20

One of the areas that my grief affected most was my relationships. Because I didn't have any family where Hannah and I lived, my friends and my community there were my only source of relational support. I have a small handful of friends and family who have faithfully stuck by my side and selflessly shown me endless demonstrations of love and support throughout this journey. I don't know if there will ever be sufficient words to express my gratitude to them or to explain how much their love and dedication has meant to me. I know I couldn't have endured this loss without their devotion to loving me through this process.

Even so, Hannah's death has strained or somehow impacted almost every relationship in my life at some point in my grief. Whether due to misguided, unhelpful words or actions, simple misunderstandings, a feeling of disconnect on one or both sides, or people walking out of my life entirely, there were a lot of times when I felt afraid to reach out and was unsure of whom I could count on.

I believe that the majority of people desperately want to help and offer comfort, and that most comments and efforts truly come from a well-meaning heart. Therefore, I don't judge or hold bitterness toward those in my life whom I felt hurt by in my grief, because I understand that grief is messy, confusing, and fragile at times. And because everyone processes loss differently, it can be very difficult for loved ones to know how to best support someone in his or her individual grief.

The relationships that were impacted the most severely for me were, unfortunately, a few of my closest ones. It was very difficult for me in situations when the approach they took in trying to support me was sometimes unhelpful and even harmful. I know it hurt them to see me suffering, and they wanted so badly to help me get out of it. Some of the hurtful comments and/or actions that continued during that season, despite my attempts to voice my needs and explain my perspective, have stuck with me.

Many of those relationships suffered through that stormy season have grown stronger now than they were before. Some, on the other hand, haven't fully recovered yet, and after many efforts and conversations, an awkward disconnect has remained that I haven't found a way to mend. It breaks my heart, but I haven't lost hope. And I still haven't lost my love and appreciation for them.

I've wrestled greatly over many relationships that I permanently lost after Hannah died. Some people in my life disappeared. Some tended to avoid me or not respond if I tried to connect or reach out to them. I had many lonely days and nights, missing those friends, trying to understand why, and trying to figure out how to make it right. As time passed, a few of those people came back into my life, and I'm grateful for those chances to reconnect. Although it was difficult at times, I chose to forgive them and embrace those friendships again because I cherish them.

If I'm honest though, I'm not completely sure that some of those relationships will ever feel quite like they did before, in regard to my feeling of safety and reliability and trust within the relationship. However, I leave that door open with hope, because I know there is always opportunity for growth and restoration. A change that occurs may be permanent, but change doesn't always have to indicate brokenness. While some people eventually did come back into my life, others did not. And grieving those lost relationships, as well as the altered ones, has been a deeply painful part of this journey for me.

In my opinion, life is too short to forfeit any opportunity to mend a wound, even if it means forgiving someone for a wound that you know has left a scar. If I want others to extend forgiveness to me for my many flaws, mistakes and shortcomings, I must also extend forgiveness and love. I can't ask for something that I myself am not willing to give. I don't want to walk around bitter and hard-hearted through life due to unfair situations and/or wounds.

We will all face that situation at some point, where we find ourselves at a crossroad and must decide whether we will allow people and the world to make us hard and bitter or whether we will choose to live in love and extend forgiveness to those who have hurt us. And I've learned to love and forgive people regardless of their status of remorse and regardless of whether it was intentional or unintentional. Forgiveness makes me a better person and clears my heart of the poison that bitterness can eventually become.

I'm grateful for my friends and family who have been there and who have tried to support me through this, no matter the difficulties. Because even in those rough patches, I can look back and see their hearts, their love, their concerns and desire to help.

We aren't meant to walk alone; I know that I couldn't have walked alone. I couldn't have done it without them, and I will be forever grateful for their selflessness and love.

*

SHARON EHLERS

Sharon's best friend Joy died in 2009 at age 52

Sharon's former fiancé John died in 2012 at age 59

For me, the relationship with Joy's husband has been the most impacted. Right now the relationship is nonexistent.

I think I am angry with him for four reasons. One, I know how upset Joy was when he decided to retire and move to Las Vegas. I don't think she felt she had much of a say in the decision. She felt like her whole world had fallen out from under her. I think that was the real start of her depression. I don't think her husband ever really understood how much his decision impacted her. In his defense, he couldn't read her mind. She needed to say something. Either way it should have been a mutual decision.

Once Joy started living in Las Vegas, gambling became her addiction. The temptation was always there. She couldn't get away from it. It was a neon sign always flashing in her face. I had hoped that when her husband knew how difficult it was for her, he would have come up with some alternatives for where they could live. It just seemed to me like he wouldn't budge. Part of me felt like maybe that was on purpose. Until I talk with him I will never know.

Two, I never understood why Joy's husband didn't do more to help her. When she had taken the pills in California and then called me in Virginia, I literally had to call and scream to convince him to get in his car and go to her. Granted, maybe after so many years of the suicide threats he had grown complacent. I just thought he could have told her family, and they all could have gotten her the help she needed. Based on how most of them had little to no idea that Joy even attempted suicide multiple times, I got the impression that he didn't say anything at all. I think they could have helped Joy or persuaded her to enter long-term rehab. It just seemed like he never went that extra step. I have tried to put myself in his shoes. I know she wasn't the easiest person to be around sometimes, but, like all of us, Joy just wanted to be loved. If he didn't love her, then he needed to move on. She deserved at least that much.

Three, I also couldn't understand what had happened on the day Joy died. I spoke with her early in the afternoon. I spoke with her husband a couple of hours later to see how she was doing. While we were on the phone, Joy walked into the house. I heard her shout "Hey there," in the background. Little did I know this would be my last interaction with her. Her husband later said that after we hung up, he left to go to the grocery store. While he was out Joy killed herself. I asked him what had been said, and he said nothing. My gut said he wasn't being honest with me, so I pulled away.

Four, if you are living with a suicidal person, why would you have guns and ammunition in your house? This makes absolutely no sense to me. Maybe the guns without the ammunition, or ammunition without the guns, but both guns and ammunition in the same place? It seems ludicrous to me. How is that keeping her safe? This made it easy for Joy to get to both. I just couldn't understand how he could let that happen. It's almost like he had handed it to her. Over time, these four things are what made me pull completely away from him. I know that someday I will talk with him, but I am just not ready yet.

John and I ended our relationship as a couple in 2008. When he died, I reached out to his mom and we shared our grief. We were always close when John and I were together. John had forbidden me to contact his mother after we broke up, and that was very hard. I think John's death brought us back in touch again. I had missed her and missed talking with her. I think it also gave her someone to talk to. She had so many questions I couldn't answer. All I knew was that the John I had fallen in love with had changed over the years. Surprisingly, she made the same comment. She felt that John had changed over the years into someone she didn't know any more. It was comforting to talk to her, but also very heartbreaking. She could have pushed me away or refused to talk with me, but she never did. If anything, John's death brought his mom back into my family's life. I am grateful we can be there for each other.

*

BONNIE FORSHEY
Bonnie's son Billy
died in 1993 at age 16

Losing my son by suicide has destroyed my life. It totally destroyed my relationship between me and my husband, because it was his medication that killed my son. I had thrown it away, and had no idea that my husband had retrieved it from the trash and put it back in the cabinet. My husband had started doing illegal drugs, and I had no idea. It was creating so much stress and so many problems at home that I believe it led to my son's suicide.

*

LAURA HABEDANK
Laura's brother Brian
died in 2010 at age 35

I think it's absolutely true that you genuinely find out who your real friends are when tragedy strikes. I had friends who I was certain would be there for me who virtually disappeared, and that hurt more than you could imagine. As if the suicide of my only sibling wasn't hard enough, I lost friends because they couldn't handle my grief or just didn't know what to say to me.

But I also gained some new friends and experienced a regeneration of friendships that had dissipated over the years; I had people I hadn't heard from in years reach out to me in unbelievably kind ways. A childhood friend whom I hadn't seen in probably ten years started calling me every week. Since I was still in my "I just can't answer the phone" phase, she left me a voicemail each time she called. She would simply say, "I know you probably don't feel like talking, and that is totally okay. Please just know that I'm thinking of you and I'm here if you want to talk; don't feel pressured to call me back, I'll completely understand if you're not ready. I love you and I'm thinking about you." I can't think of a more loving and selfless thing for a friend to do at a time like that — just to reach out to let me know I was loved but at the same time not being upset with me for not having the strength to reach back.

I had been married for six years when Brian died, and my marriage had already been struggling for a while. Just eleven months earlier we had moved to Texas from my home state of Minnesota, and the stress of that move and the loss of having my close friends around me had taken a toll on me and on my marriage, because a big part of me resented my husband for wanting that drastic move so badly. He already had friends and family here, so he had a built-in support system in place when we relocated.

I had already made wonderful friends here in Texas by the time Brian passed, which was a huge help to me because my relationship with my husband only continued to grow increasingly distant. He wanted the "old me" back and was so deeply angry at Brian for ending his own life; my husband absolutely hated how it had destroyed my spirit. As a result, I didn't feel comfortable allowing my grief to come out around him, because I didn't want to contribute to his feelings of anger at Brian; I didn't want anyone to be upset with someone I loved so much. So I did most of my crying alone, and numbed the pain at home by drinking wine and smoking weed nearly every single night.

Our relationship continued to deteriorate, and just over half a year after Brian's death we filed for divorce. It was a completely respectful, loving, and amicable divorce, and we parted as friends. A huge part of me was so relieved because the divorce was a new start for me, and I was so relieved to have the space to just work on myself and let my grief take any shape and form that it needed to without the judgment of my spouse or the pressure I put on myself to keep it together for his sake.

My parents have also since divorced. I wouldn't say that Brian's death had anything to do with it, because their marriage had been so strained for so very long but I'm sure it didn't help either. Everyone grieves differently, and I am certain that couples, when they lose a child, either grow closer together or drift farther apart. My dad has rarely spoken about my brother since Brian's death, and seems to have internalized the loss, because outwardly he doesn't seem to be grieving at all. He has even referred to me as an "only child," which is so painful because I don't consider myself an only child at all. I have a sibling. I'm a sister to a deceased brother. I haven't spoken to him about my anger about that, because I have every bit of hope that maybe he just can't express his grief. But that disparity has certainly driven another wedge in our already strained relationship. I'm sure that was hard on my mom, too.

My relationship with my mom has changed in a lot of ways, but the most pronounced way is the sense of pressure I now feel. I'm all she has left now, so I know how much she worries and panics when she can't reach me, or when I get sick, or worse, when I suffer another deep, depressive episode.

*

VICKI HECKROTH
Vicki's son Matthew
died in 2000 at age 17

I lost my friends after my son died. They all got tired of listening to me talk about Matt, and the endless rivers of tears. I was told I was no longer any fun. I didn't laugh or even smile. I wasn't interested in going out drinking or partying. I just wanted to stay home and bring awareness and prevention to suicide. Which I still do today, fifteen years later, only with a whole new group of friends, most of whom have also lost a loved one to suicide.

*

MARLISE MAGNA
Marlise's fiancé Blaine
died in 2010 at age 36

My loss caused a temporary disconnect which slowly turned into a permanent disconnect with my gran. I used to see her at least once a week when I'd take her shopping and for a meal and we'd speak via telephone often. After Blaine's death, I just withdrew and the contact became more and more infrequent. I kind of figured that she has given up on me, as she didn't phone me on my birthday for the first time ever. I kept saying I would call and go see her, but one day out of the blue she passed away. At least she had an awesome day with family, and they were all there when she died. To this day I have severe regrets over my social paralysis after my loss and not seeing my beloved gran.

*

MARCELLA MALONE
Marcella's brother Michael
died in 2014 at age 20

There is nothing like the loss of someone so close to you to affect the relationships in your life, especially with those who might not have known Michael well, or at all. The relationship between my boyfriend and me has suffered the most since Michael's death. Our pregnancy happened accidentally, and very early in our relationship. My boyfriend had a chance to meet my brother only twice, for a few hours. He didn't get a chance to know him or the strength of the bond between us. Despite that, he was the one I had to lean on. After a short week with my family, I went home to him. He was the one I woke up to after having nightmares, the one who had to pick me up off the floor when I was weak or collapsed in tears, the one who got the short end of the stick when I was angry over what I didn't know, and the one who had to meet the other half of his son's family under such terrible circumstances.

On most days my boyfriend was great about being there for me, but some days it was too much for him. We fought and barely survived as a couple a time or two. Not having a strong family or having known mine, he truly didn't understand my pain, and we took it out on each other. While we still have our down moments, surviving the biggest tragedy of my life together has made our relationship stronger than ever.

The other relationship that has suffered a lot of strain since the loss of Michael is that with my parents. We still have a strong relationship and tell each other almost everything, but it's different now. We talk little about what happened and largely leave out our emotions regarding it. I'm not comfortable sharing my feelings and struggles with them, as I know they are suffering much worse. Sometimes it's hard to leave this out, but I can't bring myself to do it. I also caught myself putting part of the blame for what happened on them, and I can't forgive myself for these thoughts. I love them too much.

*

BRIDGET PARK
Bridget's brother Austin
died in 2008 at age 14

My father and I had a lot of stress on our relationship after my brother's suicide. My mother was very comforting to me, because her older brother died by suicide as well when she was also only a teenager. My dad felt very guilty, because he thought that he was too hard on my brother and that he never cut him any slack. My parents had really high expectations for my brother and me, and we were held to a high standard at all times. Some may think that this is a good thing to have, but I don't think my brother handled it as well as I did. My dad was especially harder on my brother than he was on me, because he was two years older than me.

My dad disappeared from my life emotionally and mentally when my brother passed. When my dad was around my mother and me, he was never fully present. It was like "the lights were on but nobody's home" kind of look. My dad was also on a lot of different kinds of antidepressants after my brother passed, which often made him seem loopy and intoxicated. I think my dad took my brother's death harder than the rest of us and showed more signs of grief than the rest of us did.

It was very difficult for me to see my father in this state, but it also made me angry at him. He would miss my volleyball games or school events, because he was at work or simply forgot, whereas beforehand he had always made it a priority to go to my games and events. I know that my dad did not mean to hurt or disappoint me, but it was inevitable for me to feel this way. My dad focused so much on the fact that he lost a child, but he forgot and neglected the fact that he still has a daughter who was alive and needed her father. My mother was very sympathetic to me and tried to compensate for my dad's absence, and I really appreciate my mother in that way. This phase lasted for two to three years, and soon Dad was able to clear his head and heart. I do not resent my dad for this, because I know that he did not want to hurt me and that he was in fact hurting.

*

GRACE YOUNG
Grace's son Jack died
in 2007 on his 27th birthday

It's been hard to get my husband to release his grief. He has had a hard time dealing with guilt over the loss of our firstborn son. My husband feels that perhaps he was too hard on him, not understanding Jack's depression. We have worked hard to learn all we can about depression and suicide, in order to teach others how to recognize the signs. But with men, they feel they must be the "strong" one and hold in their feelings too much. I can tell when my husband is getting to the overflow point, and very gently try to coax the tears from him, to help him release his guilt and pain.

*

Fitting in is unnecessary.
Embrace who you are.
-NEON HITCH

*

CHAPTER TWELVE

THE FAITH

Love is the only law capable of transforming grief
into hope. -LYNDA CHELDELIN FELL

Grief has far-reaching effects in most areas of our life, including
faith. For some, our faith can deepen as it becomes a safe haven for
our sorrow. For others, it can be a source of disappointment,
leading to fractured beliefs. One commonality among the bereaved
is that faith is often altered one way or the other.

*

KAYLA ARNOLD
Kayla's uncle Tim
died in 2001 at age 34

Has my faith been impacted? When my uncle first passed, it
absolutely was! I was so mad! I felt like I could not believe in
someone who could allow my uncle to be taken from me! I know
that my uncle made the decision to end his life, but the belief in a
higher power calling him home at such a young age was something
I could not understand. I got very bitter and did lose faith in God,
and felt like I shouldn't believe in someone who allowed such
things.

159

I became very depressed, upset and hurt. I missed my uncle something fierce, and the concept of suicide was still something I just did not understand. I still could not wrap my twelve-year-old brain around why someone I loved with all my heart would willingly leave me.

But ultimately putting some faith back in God is what allowed me to heal. I am not someone who goes to church, but I believe. I believe what I want to believe about the higher power and what he does for us. But I feel like I have enough faith that I don't need to sit there and be preached to. I have my own beliefs, and I believe when it comes down to it that I have my faith and that is all I need.

Yes, when my uncle passed I lost all faith in a higher power. And that is because suicide is horrible, heartbreaking, and you cannot understand why your loved one would take his own life. And when you believe that God takes those he needs, you cannot wrap your head around why he needed your loved one or why he had to take him the way he did. That is enough to shake anyone's faith! But in the end, faith is what brought me out of my depression and gave me the strength to believe that my uncle is in a better place and at peace. He is always with me, and I know that I have one of the best guardian angels anyone could ask for.

*

EMILY BARNHARDT
Emily's friend and roommate Hannah
died in 2014 at age 20

Being a Christian and losing a loved one to suicide has brought up many unique challenges in my grief, not only in regard to my own personal faith, but also with my experience of support in the Christian community. Because of its taboo nature, I think suicide is sadly often a "hot potato" subject within the church. It's also a subject that has many different opinions and viewpoints in the context of Christianity.

In that first year after Hannah's death, my Christian faith was my only source of strength, comfort, and hope. Unfortunately, it was also one of my deepest sources of disappointment, confusion, and hurt during that time.

I know for a fact that I wouldn't have made it through this past year and a half without the Lord and His compassion for me. He has patiently walked alongside me as I've grieved, resting with me when I grew weary, reaching out His hand to help me up when I was ready to take steps forward, and never rushing or condemning me for how I was feeling. He has carried me and sustained me in every moment when I thought I couldn't go on. A bible verse that has given me great comfort since Hannah passed is Isaiah 46:4: *I am He [God], I am He who will sustain you. I have made you and I will carry you; I will sustain you and I will rescue you.*

I wish I could say that my faith in God has remained firm, unshaken and steady throughout this grief, but I would be lying if I did. I don't believe it's possible to grieve such a tragic loss and not falter or feel weak in our faith at times. It's arguably actually more common to have a complete crisis of faith at some point. It's understandable, as we are only human, and it should be received by others in our faith with compassion and patience.

It's important for every Christian to understand that a person's level of grief and how it manifests does not necessarily indicate or signify the level or quality of that person's faith. There were times in that first year of grief where my view of God seemed paradoxical. I desperately needed the reassurance that God is concretely and reliably good and safe. I needed to view Him as the God of comfort; my hope, my strength, and my rock. And I did see Him as that, because I have experienced that this is who God is and I know that He doesn't change based on our circumstances.

Nonetheless, I also found that when I looked at God, my perspective and thoughts seemed contradicting sometimes. I saw

Him as my comfort, yet I also saw Him as being the author of my discomfort. Over time, I had to acknowledge how I felt about God in regard to Hannah's suicide. After all, He did have the power to stop her from taking her life, so where was He that night? Why would He not let me help her when I was right there, when I was trying to find her, and when He knew I would have done anything and everything to save her?

I couldn't deny that unsettling flicker of anger that I felt resonate in my chest at times, or the moments where I sensed feeling unsafe with God and unsure of His goodness and His trustworthiness. It was extremely challenging and confusing at times, trying to cling in trust to the same God who I also doubted and questioned because of her death. I wrestled deeply with these thoughts. For a period of time I actually avoided communicating with God altogether on an authentic level, just to avoid having to face those painful emotions and the discomforting reality of my conflicting thoughts toward Him.

Many people sharing my Christian faith gave me their opinions and advice on why I felt the way I did, what I should be doing and thinking, what I was doing wrong in my grief process, and/or where my beliefs were faulty. Unfortunately, some of those approaches and comments were harmful for me and made me feel even more alone, conflicted, hurt, and confused in my faith.

Conversely, there were also several Christian friends who demonstrated the very love, compassion, and patience of God by showing me God's character in how they treated me. And that's how it is supposed to be; that's how we need to love one another. These friends accepted that they didn't know the answers, they didn't try to give me spiritual clichés or pat answers, they loved me and comforted me, and they empathized and accepted me in whatever state I happened to be in on that particular day. Most important, they allowed me the space to wrestle with God.

While they did gently challenge me, encourage me, and remind me of the truths that God says in the bible, they also understood that my personal relationship with God and my view of Him was an area that I needed to personally address with God alone, and only in His perfect timing. This was one of the greatest gifts of support those friends gave me, because it isn't our right to demand evidence of growth in someone else's life and/or to condemn them if they don't show what we consider to be sufficient faith. The fulfillment of the promises of God and the strength and hope we, as Christians, draw from them is through our own personal relationship with Him. It's a process that God wants to do in His own timing, because only He knows when we are ready.

Truthfully, I did feel deeply hurt by the overall Christian community during my grief, though that doesn't mean I felt hurt by every Christian. As I said, I had a handful of wonderful friends. One of God's most beautiful promises, though, is that He can take even our most painful and tragic experiences and create something good from them. I've already seen Him using what I've been through for good in many ways.

Because of the disappointment, rejection, and loneliness I felt at times within the Christian community, God has given me a fiery passion to be an advocate for those suffering within the church walls. He's given me a desire to educate and raise awareness about issues, like grief and mental health, in which I've seen misguided or unhelpful approaches and opinions. I see my experience as an opportunity not to criticize or condemn Christians, but to empower them. I want to be a voice in the issues our world faces in the context of Christianity, and empower Christians in dealing with these issues in a way that will uplift, encourage, and help those suffering.

I've heard too many stories about suffering people who have felt belittled, rejected, judged, or condemned by Christians and the church. I don't believe it's intentional; I simply believe there's a gap that needs to be bridged between certain issues that can often cause misunderstanding and misguided beliefs. When we, as Christians, come together in a way that brings life and hope and uplifting support to any person who walks through the church doors, we are a force to be reckoned with. As each of us comes together, bringing our own messy pasts and painful experiences to the table, we can learn from one another about things we haven't personally walked through. We can help educate one another, so that we can be more effective in supporting those in situations we can't relate to. We must band together, stick together, and persevere together. Without that internal effort, our unity and effectiveness will waver. Without a desire to understand one another's unique wounds, we will most likely cause more damage, rather than offering hope. And that is the desire God has put in my heart, to try to help bridge those gaps of understanding, and I'm thankful and humbled that He's already given me a voice to do so through different opportunities in my path this past year, this book being one of them.

As for my own personal faith, I'm still working on growth and healing. My belief in Christ and who He is was never shaken, but there are still wounds that need healing and areas that need to be reconstructed. There are things God is showing me, ways He is trying to help me grow, and ways He intends to deepen my faith through this grief process.

I don't have answers to all the questions I have over Hannah's death, and I've had to accept that I might never get those answers in my time here on earth. I do know Christ, however, and He has shown me throughout my life that I can trust Him and His plan, even when it doesn't make sense to me. Personally, I know that without Him I feel no hope or meaning or purpose for my life; He is what keeps me going. He is the One who gives me life, even in the darkest depths of my grief. One of the main obstacles in grieving this type of loss as a Christian is figuring out how to navigate the surplus of controversial opinions on suicide within the church and the Christian community. I know some Christians will not agree with my opinion on suicide, as is the case with discussion on any taboo subject, regardless of religion. And that's okay. However, it is a fact that I have a different perspective on this subject as a Christian, from that of another Christian per se who has never lost a close loved one to suicide and who has also not experienced that depth of darkness himself.

I think that in these situations we can benefit by listening to those who have walked paths we have not yet walked ourselves, in order to learn how we might be able to better approach that issue and be more equipped in helping people through it. I mentioned earlier in this book how I experienced a few dark nights during the first season of my grief. I can't explain that feeling of darkness that I felt on those specific nights and days. As I said, it felt like Hannah's pain had somehow transferred to me. It felt like Satan himself was hovering over me and covering me. That feeling, a feeling of terrifying and suffocating darkness, is exactly what can drive a person to take his or her own life. I can only explain it as a level of consuming darkness that no Christian, even one who is fully aware of the power of Satan, could ever begin to imagine unless he is taken to that exact level of darkness himself. It's oppression and evil that is beyond description. That is why it hurts me to hear Christians label someone who takes his own life as selfish, because I know the power of the enemy and the horrifying extent of how he can blind us.

Please hear me when I say that Christians are not to blame for the belief that suicide is selfish. It's unfortunately a common response across the board, religion or no religion, and it's a misguided and insensitive response. We assume that because a person carried out the action of taking his or her life, that person rationally made the decision to do it.

Not everyone who reads my words will share my faith, and that is entirely okay. These words are for the people who can relate to my experience and faith. I want to say that it's interesting to me that as Christians we often express our belief that the act of suicide is selfish, when the reality is this: shouldn't we as Christians actually have more understanding that suicide testifies not to a person's character, but to the level of pain and spiritual attack he was under? After all, we know how powerful Satan can be, and we know the dark deception that can so easily blind us and take over our rational minds.

I feel the need to clarify that I am not talking about someone being possessed by demons. Unfortunately, I've heard too many grieving people share with me the wounds they carry from the church, saying their loved one was possessed. I personally don't agree at all with that approach toward someone hurting. I'm also not saying that all Christians take the wrong approach; they don't. I think this is exactly why this subject is unfortunately met with defensiveness on both sides. I can only speak to my experience and the experiences I've heard from others. And I myself am a Christian, so my words have no intention other than helping those who suffer and empowering us to try to see things from a different perspective.

As Christians, we categorize things as sinful or not sinful in our minds, because that's important in how we live our lives. However, when it comes to suicide, whether it is a person currently battling it or someone having passed away from it, I wonder if our "sin categories" can sometimes unintentionally lead us first to judgment rather than discernment and compassion. Because the issue of suicide isn't about selfishness or sin; it's about deception and darkness. And we know who to blame for that...and it isn't the person who is suffering.

This is my wish for the Christian community: to reflect on how we view and approach issues such as suicide, and to make sure that the way we respond is life-giving and life-changing in a beneficial way...a way that brings hope and life.

*

CHRISTINE BASTONE
Christine's sister Elizabeth
died in 2012 at age 38

My loss made me question almost everything I have ever believed, and has also drastically changed what I believe. I clearly remember being in the library looking for books that might help me in my grief. I picked up one written by a medium, *We Are Their Heaven,* by Allison DuBois. I was always taught that mediums are a big no-no, so I put it back. But then I decided that my sister's death was causing me enough pain to read such a book anyway. And so I checked it out. I devoured it, and any other book that I can find written by a medium. I have since come to believe that it is only fake mediums who are a no-no.

After my sister died, I began to wonder what part of what I had believed was of God, and what part was only of man. One of the biggest changes is how I feel about the Bible. The original translation of the Bible is not English. Men have translated it. I believe that at least sometimes there is something missing, or maybe even inaccurate with the translation. So I no longer take it as the final authority on everything.

I also no longer oppose gay marriage. I no longer oppose gay people period, and I wish that they, along with everyone else, were welcomed with open arms at all churches.

I can no longer fathom God sending anyone to hell. I believe that Christ died to save all of us, not just a few who accept Him. I believe that hell is much more likely to frequently be here and now, and not after we die. I believe that only demons and the devil deserve hell. I do, however, believe in different levels of heaven. I also believe that we will all go through some sort of life review.

I still consider myself a Christian. I'm just no longer a fundamental Christian. I find myself being ashamed of how many other Christians treat people who are grieving and people who are survivors of a suicide attempt or of a suicide loss. I even find myself ashamed of how many Christians treat people who are different than they have been taught that people should be such as people who are divorced, living together without marriage, or are gay. In my spiritual search, I ended up finding out about how much abuse goes on in way too many churches, not that it would be acceptable for it to happen even in just one church. But even the way too many churches treat women is just awful. Not that that's the point here, but as a fellow Christian, I have been horrified and ashamed of that. Telling anyone that his or her loved one is in hell is never a Christian thing to do. Giving simplistic advice such as "All you need to do is pray and read the Bible" isn't helpful either. Judging people is no less a sin than the very things that so many Christians judge people for. And I wish they would realize that.

People are supposed to know we are Christians by our love. And too many Christians are known by their hate instead. In the support groups I belong to, I have heard so many times how much anguish is caused by many comments that too many Christians make. It makes me angry on their behalf. I just want to hug them, and tell them that not all Christians are like that.

So...yes, my faith was greatly impacted by my loss. And while I know many people won't agree with me, I think it was an impact for the better.

*

SHARON EHLERS
Sharon's best friend Joy died in 2009 at age 52
Sharon's former fiancé John died in 2012 at age 59

If anything, my faith has grown exponentially. I was born Catholic but have not been practicing my religion (i.e., going to church every week) for a few years. I didn't even consider reaching out to the Catholic church for either of these losses. It's not that I didn't think they would be helpful; it just seemed like I had to find my own way.

It was actually my spirituality that kept me going. If I hadn't been spiritual, I don't think I would have dealt very well with either John's or Joy's suicide. Their deaths would have seemed so finite. I would have had no hope of ever seeing them again. But I have learned there is more than this life. I know we are here for a purpose. I know there are even some who say we live our lives over and over again until we get it right. Any way you look at it, life doesn't end with death.

Of course when they died I was grief-stricken. Just because you believe there is more to life doesn't mean that you don't grieve. What helped me, though, was knowing they were okay, that they were in a place where they were safe, protected, and loved. That their pain was finally gone.

In my own curiosity, I started reading books about the afterlife by Sylvia Browne, John Edward, and other authors. I wanted to know if something different happened to someone who committed suicide. As a Catholic I had always believed in heaven and life after death, but there was always that fire and brimstone about what happens to people who sin. Was suicide considered sinful? I didn't think so, because I believe that God loves everyone. Joy and John were good people who had hit a few big bumps in their lives. God would never turn His back on them. I guess all the reading I did was to confirm that they were going to make it. That they weren't stuck in some purgatory place or wandering the earth because they had taken their own lives.

I guess you really don't give it much thought until it hits close-to-home. After my maternal and paternal grandmothers both died, I had very vivid dreams of both of them. At first I was just blown away because of how real it had seemed after I woke up. Over time,

I realized this was their way of giving me the message that they were okay. Since my grandmothers' deaths, I have had similar experiences too numerous to count. It made me realize that our loved ones are always with us. I have likened it to their sitting around watching us like we are on TV. Heavenly TV. Channel Cloud Nine. They are probably laughing and crying with us as we journey through life. So when Joy died, I knew it wasn't the end. I knew she was around me by the smell of her perfume. I knew John was around me by the songs on the radio. Their deaths actually strengthened my faith in God. It confirmed that we don't just die and that's the end. We move on to something more wonderful than we could imagine. Knowing there is life after death has helped me to not be consumed by their deaths. It has helped me to not be afraid to die. When you are not afraid to die, you live more fully, or at least try to. As Mark Twain once wrote, "The fear of death follows from the fear of life. A man who lives fully is prepared to die at any time."

In some ways, Joy's and John's deaths have helped me to live more fully, appreciate the beauty of life around me, and cherish my family beyond measure. I feel blessed to know there is something more waiting for us.

*

BONNIE FORSHEY

Bonnie's son Billy

died in 1993 at age 16

It certainly has changed my way of thinking. At my son's funeral, our pastor stood in front of hundreds of his friends and told them all to never opt for suicide, or they would end up in hell like my son. I have not been back to a church since then.

*

LAURA HABEDANK
Laura's brother Brian
died in 2010 at age 35

The issue of faith is kind of a tricky one for me. I was raised going to church, and became increasingly active in my youth group in junior high and high school. However, the older I got and the more I learned about all kinds of other religions, the less sense *any* of them made to me. I decided years ago that I don't believe we were created by a "heavenly being in the sky." I do, however, believe that we are all made of energy and are connected, and that after death a part of us lives on in some form.

Some of the more hurtful things I've heard numerous times since Brian's suicide include: "It was God's will," or "God needed another angel," or "He's with Jesus now," or "God doesn't give you more than you can handle." I wish that people wouldn't be so quick to assume that I share their beliefs, because those statements did me more harm than good. And after my father attempted suicide in 1995, a born-again Christian friend of mine, instead of simply saying, "I'm sorry that happened, I hope he's okay now," he chose to proclaim to me that my dad would be spending an eternity burning in hell for committing the "ultimate sin." To date, that is still one of the most uncaring and heartless things anyone ever said to me. I don't see the point of saying something like that to another human being who is hurting.

While I don't believe in the idea of heaven or hell, I do believe that our spirits continue in some shape or form. I've felt that way for quite some time, even long before Brian's death. But just six weeks after he died, I had the most amazing experience, and I'm positive that Brian visited me in a dream. In this dream, Mom and I were in some house, I believe it was supposed to be Brian's place, although everything looked so different. I heard his voice, very groggy, as though he were just waking up. He was calling my name, saying "Laura...., Laura....it's Brian." I was frantically looking around, thinking there was no way I could have just heard what I thought I heard. I ran down the stairs, and as I approached the last few steps I saw Brian walking toward me. For some reason he was carrying an oxygen tank and had a breathing tube going to his nose. I sat down on the bottom few steps with Mom sitting just a few steps behind me. As Brian stood on the floor next to the staircase, he took both my hands in his. I thought to myself, "There is no way this is happening; could he really be here with us now?" I glanced up at Mom and cried as I asked her, "Mom, what is happening?" I needed to see if she was hearing and seeing what I was, and she assured me that she was. However, I sensed from her that it didn't mean that he was alive. I looked at Brian again and he looked really good. He looked so peaceful and rested and happy. He had that pink glow back in his cheeks, and his eyes told me he was okay. I asked him how he was and he said, "I'm all right now. I was cured the moment I passed away. I love you very much and I miss you." I told him that I loved him and missed him too, and hugged him and cried. I kept looking at Mom to see if she was hearing it, and she kept assuring me that she was. But she stayed there quietly next to me and just watched and listened, as if she knew that this moment with Brian was meant just for me.

Then Mom and I were saying our goodbyes downstairs to Brian as if we were leaving his place like other times before. Mom asked, "Are you going to be okay? What are you going to do now?" He said, "I'm good. I'm going to just run out for a bit." He had a cup of coffee in one hand and reached for his car keys with the other, as if he were truly only going to hop into his red Saturn and go for a drive. That's the thing last I remember before waking up. I woke up feeling so peaceful and grateful that I'd had that dream. I believed then, and still believe today, that it was my brother reaching out to let me know that he wasn't suffering anymore. It was the most unbelievably moving experience of my life.

Brian wasn't a religious person either. I chose the beautiful, non-religious writings to be included in the funeral service. We also chose to include a poem that Grandpa Ralph had written not long before his own death in 2003:

> If you happen to think of me
> Remember how I used to be.
> And when, while you're pausing,
> After I am laid to rest,
> Take a moment to recall
> That of me that was best.

I thought this poem particularly fitting, as I want Brian to be remembered for his life and his loving spirit, not for the manner in which he died, because there was so much more to him that those who loved him were lucky enough to experience. And there is not a single part of me that will ever believe there is a god out there somewhere who sent my brother's soul to some kind of eternal, fiery hell for giving up.

*

VICKI HECKROTH
Vicki's son Matthew
died in 2000 at age 17

My faith went by the wayside and had gotten lost sometime prior to my son's death. After his death I began to lean heavily on what faith I had left, and it has blossomed in full bloom now. I don't honestly believe I would have survived without my faith. It consumes most of my life now. Knowing that one day I will be reunited with both my son (suicide) and my mother (car accident), as well as my grandparents, whom I loved dearly, is what gets me through many days.

*

MARLISE MAGNA
Marlise's fiancé Blaine
died in 2010 at age 36

Yes! In a positive way! When Blaine died I was not really a believer, for lack of a better word. I was more spiritual and just said "Yes, there is a God," but that's that. His mom had arranged a Christian memorial service for him, but I don't believe he was a Christian at his passing. When I was in the hospital after his death, pastors tried to reach out to me, but I would not even see them, and got very irritated by their concern for a stranger. About two years later I started dating a pastor. He never forced the issue, and one day we just got to discussing Jesus, when *bam*, his statements made sense and he could back them up with hard evidence. Subsequently, I got saved, enrolled to study theology, and have since stepped into ministry and counseling. I wish my faith could show others that there IS hope and life after a loss. Also that it would give people more strength after their loss, because we will see our loved ones again. My faith has been my strength ever since.

*

MARCELLA MALONE
Marcella's brother Michael
died in 2014 at age 20

I have always been a nondenominational Christian. Growing up, I always attended church, was in youth group, worked in the church nursery, taught children's church, etc. The farther I got into college, the less I attended church or did anything with this aspect of my life. After Michael's death, I found great comfort in thoughts of heaven and the prospect of seeing him again one day. This brought me to finding a church to attend that was near my new home, and making the decision to raise my child in a church. While my relationship with my faith was strengthened, I have also found that I am more skeptical of what I hear, am more emotional toward certain topics, and have to deal with my anger toward God for taking away my brother. My faith has been a rollercoaster since Michael's death, with my comfort always being in heaven and my belief that suicide does not keep you out of it.

*

JULIE MJELVE
Julie's husband Cameron
died in 2011 at age 42

My faith has indeed been impacted by my loss. Fortunately, I can say that it has been deepened. It has caused me to question my beliefs in God, especially why God would allow this to happen, why he didn't "save" my husband and find Cameron the help he needed. I make my guesses. My husband was hurting, and perhaps God allowed it as a way to set him free from his pain.

At my husband's funeral I had them play the song "Amazing Grace." My chains are gone, I've been set free. I could see that my husband's mental illness was destroying him. So at least now he's in a place where there is no more pain.

I still hurt, but God can also help me through that pain and give me the strength to make it through another day. Cameron's tombstone says "Earth has no sorrow that heaven cannot heal." There is another song that has helped me find meaning. It's called "Blessings," by Laura Story. The song has wonderful lyrics, and some of the most powerful for me are "What if your blessings come through raindrops, what if your healing comes through tears, what if a thousand sleepless nights are what it takes to know you're near? What if trials of this life are your mercies in disguise?" This has been a very difficult time for me. But I have found that I am a different person. I think I'm stronger in many different ways. I stand up more for myself. I speak out more for others. I've learned that instead of praying for God to take away the pain and the difficulties I now experience as a result of the loss of my husband (which He never answers!), I now pray that God would provide for me whatever the resources I need for the particular difficulty, whether it be finances, a meal, a shoulder to cry on, words of comfort. These He does answer. And as a result, I've learned how to trust in God more. What I wish Christians would do more of in their approach and support of the bereaved is to act more. Words and cards are nice, but the best way to show your love and God's love for others is to serve them. It's traditional to make a meal, and it is absolutely appreciated, but I would recommend to go a step farther. Do some dishes. Do some laundry. Help with groceries. I just read about a family from a farming community that experienced a loss, and the news report stated how the whole family community is coming together to make sure the crops get harvested. To me, this shows God's love far more than patting me on the shoulder and telling me my husband is in heaven now.

*

BRIDGET PARK
Bridget's brother Austin
died in 2008 at age 14

My faith increased drastically when my brother passed. I was only twelve when he passed, and before his death I had never had any traumatic events that I really needed to lean on my faith for.

I believe that my brother is in heaven and that his spirit is with us every day. I am Catholic, so only about a decade ago suicide was still considered to be a mortal sin, meaning that one can go to hell for this. I do not agree with this teaching, but thankfully the church has reformed it. At my brother's funeral our priest spoke of forgiveness and the unconditional love that God has for us, which was very comforting to hear and get reassurance that my brother will go to heaven.

Despite this, there was a phase when I was angry at God and did not understand why He couldn't save my brother from his terrible mistake. He performs medical miracles every day, and I struggled with the question of why he did not save my brother and keep him alive. I was angry that my brother was not worthy of God's grace because God did not step in and save his life.

I became very angry and resentful toward God, and I questioned His ability. I questioned whether there is a point when science overrules miracles, and if there was any possible way for God to do anything to help my brother. Since Austin shot himself and it happened so fast, was God not prepared to save him, or was the wound too severe? I was very indifferent to my faith at this point, and ignored it for about a year.

I finally came to peace with this about a year ago, and my faith has grown ever since. I am not as religious as I was when I was living back home with my parents, but my faith has grown and I am relying on it more now that I am an adult.

*

GRACE YOUNG
Grace's son Jack died
in 2007 on his 27th birthday

My faith has only been made stronger by the loss of my son. I do not blame God for his death. I blame mental illness, and our lack of education in recognizing the signs of suicide. I am so thankful that I have God in my life, a loving church family, and a strong belief that my son is in heaven, safe in Jesus' arms, and that one day our family will be reunited.

*

Start where you are. Use what you have. Do what you can.
ARTHUR ASHE

*

CHAPTER THIRTEEN

OUR HEALTH

Health is a state of complete physical, mental, and social well-being, and not merely the absence of disease or infirmity. WORLD HEALTH ORGANIZATION

As our anatomical and physiological systems work in tandem with our emotional well-being, when one part of our body is stressed, other parts become compromised. Has your grief affected your physical health?

*

EMILY BARNHARDT
Emily's friend and roommate Hannah
died in 2014 at age 20

I've always heard how emotional stress and trauma can take a toll on our physical bodies. I'm convinced of this, because I've experienced the common physical ailments that can be brought on by emotional stress in times of my life, including, but not limited to, stomach issues, headaches, backaches, nausea, chest pain, and fatigue. But in my grief, I experienced just how severely emotional trauma can realistically impact the physical body.

In August 2014, three months after Hannah passed, the immediate shock dissipated and the reality of her absence began to hit. My world was spinning and moving faster than I could keep up; I was overwhelmed by the grief and by the events of dealing with her belongings, moving to a new apartment, going back to work, beginning another semester of college classes, and having my volunteer commitments starting up for the year again. I was blindly stumbling through each day, simply trying to withstand the pace.

It was also around that time when I noticed that my support system had diminished somewhat. I felt extremely alone, depressed, and began experiencing panic attacks from the overwhelming anxiety and stress. My doctor wasn't surprised when I suddenly developed shingles out of nowhere; she told me it was likely that the grief and stress had caused or contributed to it. I was emotionally unraveling, and the pain of shingles felt excruciating at times.

The shingles healed slowly over time, but come December my health started declining again. I began having random bouts of nausea and vomiting, chest pain, and terrible acid reflux. In January I went to a gastrointestinal doctor and began going through a myriad of unpleasant tests and procedures in search of an answer. When he couldn't find any cause for my symptoms after a month, he gave up trying and told me not to come back.

My health began declining more and more, and I started battling crippling fatigue, headaches, dizziness, intense neck pain, and other random ailments. There were many days when I couldn't get out of bed due to the unbelievable fatigue. Sometimes I didn't even have the energy to sit upright on the couch to watch TV, let alone get dressed and go anywhere.

I started getting random conditions and infections that were unrelated except for the common denominator of some type of internal inflammation. I developed plantar fasciitis in my foot and had to undergo painful steroid injections every week. It seemed I had a new condition every week; one week it was a harmless skin condition, the next week a bladder infection, the next week I was in the emergency room for fainting at work, and so on. I ended up in the emergency room multiple times, actually, one of which was for a severely deep skin infection which then began to spread into my lymphatic system. I was under anesthesia twice in two months, getting blood drawn every week, volleying between four and five different specialized doctors regularly. I was forced to take medical leave from my college that semester due to missing so many classes for appointments, tests, procedures, or feeling too sick to get out of bed. My health had gone absolutely haywire and none of the dots seemed to connect.

These health issues occurred over a period of four to five months, then began to dissipate slowly, for reasons I still don't know. Looking back, especially in writing this, I'm bewildered over the chaos of that health crisis. It amazes me how linked our physical health is to our mental health, to the extent that emotions can wreak that much havoc on one's body. That's why it is so crucial to learn to listen to your body, especially in grief; listen to what it needs, honor your limits, take care of yourself, and prioritize keeping yourself healthy.

The worse my health was, the harder it was for me to handle the grief, the stressors and the emotions. It's a correlative relationship: our physical condition affects our mental state and our mental state affects our physical condition. Neglecting one will also harm the other, because grief can manifest in either form. For example, unintentionally bottling up the emotions can push the grief to manifest physically. Grief has to go somewhere; we cannot make it disappear, no matter how hard we try. It's like an old leaky pipe. We can try to plug one hole, but another will always appear.

That's why, in order to best take care of ourselves in our grief, we must prioritize both our health and our emotions. We need both entities to be healthy in order for us to possibly persevere through this type of pain.

*

CHRISTINE BASTONE
Christine's sister Elizabeth
died in 2012 at age 38

It didn't really affect my health. I already had chronic fatigue syndrome for a long time before my loss. That being said, grief is very exhausting. I think it has increased the exhaustion that I already feel on a daily basis. And of course it certainly hasn't improved my health any.

*

SHARON EHLERS
Sharon's best friend Joy died in 2009 at age 52
Sharon's former fiancé John died in 2012 at age 59

After Joy died there was such a deep sadness. My whole body felt so heavy. My mind was in a daze all the time. I could cry at the drop of a hat. I felt so empty. I couldn't describe to anyone how I felt. I just know I didn't feel like myself anymore. Luckily for me, I had been receiving Reiki energy healing for a while to help myself decompress from a stressful job. After Joy died, one of the first things I did was make an appointment for a Reiki session. I knew it would keep me physically and spiritually balanced. I also tried to make sure that I practiced Reiki self-care to keep from getting sick.

I know it's common for people who are grieving to be more prone to illness or accidents, and with three children I just couldn't go there. I honestly think that because of the Reiki I stayed healthier physically and spiritually. That doesn't mean I had it together emotionally. I most certainly did not. I went through all the ups and downs every griever goes through. I was sad, then very sad, then very, very sad. Some days were okay; most days were tough. I was hungry; I wasn't hungry. I could sleep; then I couldn't. For a long while I couldn't close my eyes at night because I didn't want to replay the picture I had created in my head of Joy killing herself. Eventually that went away, but I still couldn't sleep. I forced myself to go out for evening walks. The fresh air helped a lot with feeling and sleeping better. I found that walking gave me a safe place to plug in my earphones, listen to music, and cry my way through the neighborhood. It was the only place other than my car or in bed at night where I could really cry. When you are working you have to walk around with that "I am fine" smile plastered on your face even if you don't feel fine. Walking gave me the freedom to feel how I wanted to feel. Being a single mom forced me to make sure I didn't fall apart. I showed my children my emotional grief, but I made sure I did what I could to take care of myself physically and spiritually.

The physical symptoms were much more intense with John. It was hard to imagine that it would be tougher than what I had felt with Joy, but I saw him as my one true love in life. After he died I felt like my heart had actually broken into a million pieces. It literally ached inside my body to the point where I thought I was going to have a heart attack. Sometimes it was hard to breathe. I convinced myself I was on the verge of a heart attack, so I went to the doctor. Everything was normal he said. So it appeared like the grief was creating this pain. It was like someone had gone in and pulled out both my heart and soul in one fell swoop. I felt completely empty and drained, like a piece of me was missing.

Again I turned to Reiki. It took me to a place where my body felt peaceful. I knew that my grief was manifesting itself in physical symptoms. I needed to stop that, so I made sure I practiced Reiki every day. It is amazing how much better you function when your body doesn't feel like it is about to fall apart. In some ways it also opened up the emotional floodgates. Since I knew there wasn't anything wrong with me physically, it brought the emotions to the forefront. So I just faced it head-on. I allowed it to come and go, allowed myself to cry in front of my children, allowed myself to feel the emotions. I just vowed to let it go. I know that releasing those emotions helped in ways I probably don't even know. I have to say that I am thankful for Reiki, my own spirituality, and the role they both played in helping me avoid physically falling apart.

*

BONNIE FORSHEY
Bonnie's son Billy
died in 1993 at age 16

My health has deteriorated. I have been progressively getting worse. It started out with depression and led to many autoimmune diseases.

*

LAURA HABEDANK
Laura's brother Brian
died in 2010 at age 35

In the five years since Brian's death I have gained forty pounds, and honestly I don't feel healthy at all. My energy level is still poor, though I do get out for the occasional hike. I'm completely aware that my self-soothing by way of a lot of wine and pretty much anything and everything that I feel like eating has caused the decline in my physical health. I know something needs to change, but for now I just don't have the energy to do much about it.

It angers me when people preach to me about depression and how "if you'd just eat better and exercise, it would help you so much with your mood." At my healthiest, I was running fifty to sixty miles a week, eating well, I consumed no caffeine or alcohol yet I was deeply depressed, feeling suicidal and self-injuring multiple times a day. I'd never argue that exercise and a healthy diet aren't good for you, because they absolutely are, but they aren't a treatment for clinical depression. Even at that healthy weight and having enough energy to get up at 5:30 a.m. and run twelve miles before work, I still hated my body, felt insecure and hopeless. It wasn't until I was put on medication that I noticed an improvement in my mood. That was fifteen years ago, and I'm still on medication today, though I go to my psychiatrist multiple times a year to stay on top of the dosage.

I recall Brian and I having a conversation before he died about physical health in relation to depression, too. In 2004, Brian entered his first bodybuilding competition, and I was so impressed with all his hard work. In addition to working full time he was also going to school, had a part-time weekend job, and did all his training for the competition alone. He studied up on it a great deal and was so impressively diligent about sticking to a strict diet and lifting routine, and his physique changed in a startling way. He confided in me that he had found himself over-exercising often as a way to distract himself from his feelings of depression, and it became an unhealthy addiction of sorts. I shared with him that I felt the same way about all my running; I began to use it as a coping mechanism that became an obsession. In addition to all the cutting I was doing, each time I was feeling depressed or anxious I would throw on my running shoes and go run anywhere from six to nine miles…multiple times a day! I realized I was using it as a distraction from my feelings. It made me realize that when you're that depressed, anything can become an unhealthy pastime if abused. I reached an unhealthily low weight, and it concerned me and it concerned those who loved me. Sadly, I've now swung back to the other side of the pendulum and am painfully aware that my body isn't so happy with the choices I've been making for myself lately; that's something I definitely need to work on.

*

VICKI HECKROTH
Vicki's son Matthew
died in 2000 at age 17

Since the loss of my son I have been diagnosed with major clinical depression, rheumatoid arthritis, fibromyalgia, spinal stenosis, osteoporosis, posttraumatic stress disorder, anxiety, and degenerative disc disease. Prior to his death, I was completely healthy. I truly believe that Matt's death had a part in causing my health problems.

*

MARLISE MAGNA
Marlise's fiancé Blaine
died in 2010 at age 36

It has affected my health as well as my appearance in a major way. Appearance-wise, after Blaine passed, I lost a lot of weight and kept changing my look. I went from short hair to long, to shaving it all off and getting many piercings. Now I am a bit more "normal" and no more piercings and bald head for me. I guess I was trying to find myself or the authentic me. My identity was always defined by my partner so I felt adrift and lost in the world.

Health-wise, I did have pre-existing conditions before his passing, but they increased substantially after my loss. I developed a blood sugar problem, causing me to gain weight again. My chronic pain disorder sent my pain levels through the roof. I am constantly ill with something. The biggest problem I've had since my partner's passing is that I suffer from severe insomnia. I cannot take sleeping tablets, as I sleepwalk and drink more pills in my sleep. They also paralyze my breathing. Nighttime is terror time for me. I have this saying that "4 a.m. knows all my secrets...."

*

MARCELLA MALONE
Marcella's brother Michael
died in 2014 at age 20

For the first year or so after my brother's death, I became less interested in being healthy and getting into shape. I had spent the previous year working on this and was in the best shape and at the lowest weight I had been since middle school, despite being seven months pregnant. After Michael's death I felt no motivation to continue and had become rather lazy. Through the first year after my son's birth I gained twenty-five pounds. In the last month or so I have just gotten back to getting healthy again, but I am barely able to run a mile. With his birthday coming up in less than two weeks, I catch myself slipping back into a rut. I need to keep reminding myself to change before it causes more health problems for the sake of being around for my child. Grief definitely makes health a larger struggle for me.

*

GRACE YOUNG
Grace's son Jack died
in 2007 on his 27th birthday

I have not experienced a change in my physical health since losing my son to suicide. I try hard to concentrate on remaining healthy, as I care for my eighty-three-year-old mother, who cannot walk well and needs a lot of help.

*

BLESSINGS
BY LAURA STORY

What if your blessings
come through raindrops

What if your healing
comes through tears

And what if a thousand
sleepless nights are what
it takes to know you're near

*

CHAPTER FOURTEEN

THE QUIET

Heavy hearts, like heavy clouds in the sky, are best relieved by the letting go of a little water.
-ANTOINE RIVAROL

The endless void left in our loved one's absence remains day and night. When our minds are free from distractions there is a moment when sorrow fills the void, threatening to overtake us, unleashing the torrent of tears. For some, that moment happens during the day, for others it comes at night. What time is hardest for you?

*

KAYLA ARNOLD
Kayla's uncle Tim
died in 2001 at age 34

I don't really have one time of day that is worse than any other. For me it's more when something reminds me of my uncle like a song, a smell, a memory, or anything at all. Sometimes football season can be emotional for me. We are both diehard University of Michigan fans, and so sometimes when watching the games it's a little bittersweet. I get my passion for football and Michigan from him, and the fact that he isn't here to share those moments, games, and amazing experiences with me is hard. Last year when my mom, my boyfriend, and I went to the Big House (the stadium's nickname) for my first-ever University of Michigan game, it was really hard, because I know that if my uncle were still here he would have been there! There are so many things that remind me of him, and those are the times I have more difficulty with than a certain time of the day. It's the memories that come with the important and great moments that hit you the most. It's the daily little things that hurt a lot, but my uncle missing the big stuff is painful too. It isn't a certain time of day that is bothersome; it's just the little things, the reminders, the things I wish he were there for, the conversations I wish I could have, or the people I'd like him to meet. Those are the painful and hard times, those are the moments that make my day stop in its tracks, and those are the times I miss him more than normally.

*

CHRISTINE BASTONE
Christine's sister Elizabeth
died in 2012 at age 38

For a long time my hardest time of day was between 7:30 p.m. until around 10 p.m. You see, my parents called me a little after 8 p.m. on that fateful day that I learned Liz had died. And so any time the phone rang around that same time, I would automatically panic. This went on for at least a year. Thankfully, ever since a good friend of mine starting calling me a lot around that same time, the panic lessened a bit. Since I knew it was likely my friend who was calling, I was able to relax to a large degree. But I still feel at least a twinge of fear every time the phone rings during the evening.

*

SHARON EHLERS
Sharon's best friend Joy died in 2009 at age 52
Sharon's former fiancé John died in 2012 at age 59

When I first learned about Joy's suicide, nighttime was the worst for me. For some reason I was afraid to close my eyes, because I didn't want to imagine how she had killed herself. For a while I kept playing it over and over in my head, even though I had been in another state when it happened. I just kept walking myself through what I created in my own mind as the events. I just kept seeing it over and over again. It was hard to sleep those first few weeks and months.

After the initial shock wore off and I thought rationally about what had happened, it became easier to stop myself from going down that path in my head. After receiving so many signs from her, I began to use my quiet time at night to talk with her. The visions of her death slowly subsided and disappeared. I began to dream of her doing what she loved to do, like shopping. I remember saying to her in my dream, "But Joy, you are dead. Why are we buying all this stuff?" and she just looked at me and smiled. Maybe it was her way of getting me to think of her and all the positive memories we had shared. Whatever the reason, nighttime eventually stopped being the hardest time for me.

With John, every moment of every day was the hardest. My brain couldn't stop thinking about him. I went to work and tried to get through the day, but he was always with me. I think that because I had loved him from the depths of my soul, the grief just became a part of my DNA.

I found that when I was alone I was able to release the pain through my tears. I yearned for the alone time, because being around people all day at work just made it much harder. Work became a symbol for things that were really not important, like all

191

the meetings for no reason and all the government programs that were doomed to fail anyway. I wanted to say, "We are talking about the same stuff over and over again, day after day, year after year. Nothing is being accomplished. In the bigger scheme of life, all this is so unimportant. Loving the people who mean the most to us is what really matters. If we just worked like it was our last day, we might actually get something done. I am not sure I can sit here in this stupid place with all these stupid people anymore." This is the kinder version. What I really wanted to say was, "Someone I loved just blew their brains out. Why are we talking about all this crazy stuff in yet another stupid meeting?" I wanted to shout it at the top of my lungs. I would have loved to see the expressions on their faces. Most of them would probably have agreed.

But I held back. Holding back made it tougher to be there. Grieving and working just made it more evident how much unhappiness my job was bringing into my life. There had to be something out there which meant much more than forty to sixty hours a week of this mess. I was wasting so much time. Too many years in the same endless mess. Life was short. Life was precious. Life needed to have meaning. That's why being at work during the day after John died was definitely one of the hardest times for me.

*

BONNIE FORSHEY
Bonnie's son Billy
died in 1993 at age 16

Every day is hard. The holidays and anniversary dates are agonizing. I have learned to go on, but it is not easy. I miss him on Mother's Day, his birthday, holidays. There are constant reminders everywhere. The hardest part of the day is between 6:30 and 7 p.m. That is the time when my son ended his life. I remember everything vividly and live it over and over again. From 7 p.m. on, it was a nightmare, as they tried to bring him back. I can still hear them telling me that he didn't make it, and I can hear my screams, never-ending screams.

*

LAURA HABEDANK
Laura's brother Brian
died in 2010 at age 35

In the beginning, mornings were the hardest for me mostly because I was always so tired from night after night of restless sleep. But also because it was so hard to drag myself out of bed knowing full well that I didn't have the emotional fortitude to focus on work, or even be around people at all. It was far easier when I could just stay home, zone out in front of the TV, or cry myself to sleep multiple times a day and just pretend the rest of the world had stopped to wait for me.

Each time I left the apartment was a brutal reminder that everyone, and everything, would continue to keep on moving whether I was ready or not. I hated the fact that each sunrise meant I was moving farther and farther away from the last time I saw my brother. The evenings weren't quite as bad, because I was just exhausted from fighting through my sadness all day. And by the time I'd been home from work for an hour, I was typically three glasses of wine and two sleeping pills into my evening regimen. By that time I would just wait for my body to relax into the chemically-induced sleep that was sure to come.

I've noticed that now there isn't really a time of day that's harder than others; the grief can creep up on me quickly at any time and it's usually triggered by something that reminds me of Brian. It could be seeing a car that looks just like his, hearing a song that he loved, or driving past a restaurant he loved. Honestly, having spent thirty-five years of my life with him, there isn't much out there that doesn't remind me of him. I see and hear reminders everywhere. But there isn't a single day that passes when he isn't on my mind.

*

VICKI HECKROTH
Vicki's son Matthew
died in 2000 at age 17

Monday evenings are the hardest. My son passed away on November 6, which was a Monday, at 8:08 p.m. I will never forget that day and time. The number eight is very significant to me, as is the number three. Matthew was born on 8-3-83 and weighed eight pounds, three ounces. He died at 8:08 p.m.

*

MARLISE MAGNA
Marlise's fiancé Blaine
died in 2010 at age 36

Definitely the evenings. I never battled sleeping, but since Blaine died I have become an insomniac. Sometimes I'm awake seventy-two hours on end before getting a few hours of fitful, nightmare-filled sleep. I can't really say why, although I suspect it's posttraumatic stress disorder as diagnosed. Sadly, it's only gotten worse and worse. The worst of the worst for me is usually between 2 a.m. and 4 a.m. They say night is always darkest before the daylight breaks, and that's exactly how I experience it: a pitch black void filled with deafening silence.

*

MARCELLA MALONE
Marcella's brother Michael
died in 2014 at age 20

The hardest time of day for me since Michael's loss has definitely been night. It's the time of day when my mind wonders and brings out the questions. Why? What if? What could have been? I begin to remember all of our memories and the plans we had made as siblings for our future and wonder how my life is going to be different without him in them.

It's too quiet after everyone is in bed, and it brings up a lot of sadness for me. Some nights are better than others, but in the last year and a half it hasn't gotten much easier for me. The hardest part is when I let my mind wander too much prior to falling asleep, because then the nightmares I had in the beginning come back. I see Michael with the shotgun under his chin. I see the tears in his eyes as he pulls the trigger. I see the gore of what happens as the bullet hits him and his lifeless body remains. At this point I wake up in panic and tears. I get my son out of his crib and bring him to my bed and just watch as he sleeps, remembering I have something to live for. Luckily, these occurrences have decreased from every time I shut my eyes to once every couple of weeks. The nights have gotten easier, but the struggle is still very much there.

*

JULIE MJELVE
Julie's husband Cameron
died in 2011 at age 42

Bedtime is the hardest time of day for me. The kids keep me quite busy during the day and evening, but when everything has settled and it's time to head to that lonely, empty bed, that's when I struggle. I look at the duvet cover, which we picked out as a

SURVIVING LOSS BY SUICIDE

wedding present, and it's just such a reminder that not only is he gone, but I am alone. My dreams for our future together are gone. I would like to buy a new duvet cover and start over, redecorate the bedroom, but since he's been gone money has been tight, and I just can't afford it. Also, it upsets me to think that I *need* to give it away, as we chose it because we both really loved it. I still love the design of it, and it makes me angry to feel like I can't enjoy it, the way I should be able to. So, bedtime is my hardest time of day.

*

BRIDGET PARK
Bridget's brother Austin
died in 2008 at age 14

The hardest time of day for me is when I am sitting in class or I am not completely occupied doing something. Then I then think about my brother's suicide. I visualize his dead body on the floor next to the gun he had stuck into his mouth. I am forever haunted by this image, because no matter how hard I try to forget it, it pops into my head at the most random times. When this happens, I feel a surge of heat rushing through my body and tears in my eyes. Then I try to think about something happy, or happy memories of my brother.

It saddens me that the way I think and remember my brother is this image, so I try to condition my brain to replace it with a better memory and image of him.

*

CHAPTER FIFTEEN

OUR FEAR

The oldest and strongest emotion of mankind is fear, and the oldest and strongest kind of fear is fear of the unknown. -H. P. LOVECRAFT

Fear can cut like a knife and immobilize us like a straitjacket. It whispers to us that our lives will never be the same, our misfortunes will manifest themselves again, and that we are helpless. How do we control our fear, so it doesn't control us?

*

KAYLA ARNOLD
Kayla's uncle Tim
died in 2001 at age 34

What am I afraid of? My biggest fear is to lose someone close to me to suicide again! That pain is something I NEVER want to suffer through again! It's been fourteen years since my uncle ended his life, and I struggle with it daily. Some days are better than others, but there isn't a day that he doesn't cross my mind and I don't wish he were here. I do not ever want to have to hurt and miss someone that way again! The pain your heart feels when your loved one ends his or her life is unbearable, and the daily pain and suffering of missing them while knowing that they chose to leave you is heartbreaking. Yes, over time you learn to live your life with the pain, but some days that pain is still uncontrollable.

I think another fear would be that another loved one or friend commits suicide and I failed to help them. I have become a strong advocate for suicide prevention and education. I believe that every teacher, parent, grandparent, sibling, coworker, or even every random stranger should know the signs of suicide and be able to reach out that helping hand to someone who needs it. I have reached out to many people whom I saw on social media making suicidal comments, and I have been able to help save lives by knowing the warning signs and being willing to help someone.

Whenever I get an opportunity to educate, I do. Whether it is writing a paper, posting on social media or just talking to someone, I take that opportunity and I educate. Because ignoring suicide is not going to save a life. Prevention, education, and action are what saves lives! And the only way to save a life is to know what to look for, and when you see it, don't turn a blind eye. Take action and try to help that person. You never know when a simple, "Hey, how are you?" can completely change someone's life.

*

EMILY BARNHARDT
Emily's friend and roommate Hannah
died in 2014 at age 20

Fear is something I struggle with in all areas of my life, and one of my deepest fears is losing the people I love. I've lost other loved ones in my life before Hannah, so I've always been very aware of how short life can be and that we're never guaranteed that we will forever be with those we love. The fear of someone I love dying is an enormous fear for me, and losing Hannah opened an entirely new depth of it in me, because the pain of losing her is beyond my ability to even put into words. It terrifies me to think of going through this pain again and losing someone else I dearly love, and it terrifies me knowing that this type of nightmare can suddenly begin in a split second when you get that call or hear those words that your loved one is gone.

Since Hannah's death, I've noticed a significant increase of this immense fear that takes me to irrational, paranoid moments more often than I like to admit. There are moments, sometimes for no apparent reason at all, when I get hit with this random immense wave of panic, thinking that something has happened to one of my friends or family members. It's intensified if I can't reach them. It's often completely irrational and unjustifiable, as half the time there's no red flag indicating a need for concern, so I don't know what triggers those random moments when I panic about the safety of someone. All I know is that I'll suddenly get terrified and have a desperate need to know that a certain person is okay. Thankfully, my loved ones have been compassionate and understanding toward this heightened fear I've had, and they've been patient with me in the times I've randomly sent them a frantic, worried text out of the blue. They won't make a big deal about it; they simply respond reassuringly that everything is okay, fully understanding where the anxiety is truly coming from. Sometimes I approach it jokingly now and will just say, "Just having an irrational anxious moment, and need to know you're okay." I've appreciated their patience and understanding with me and the intense fear this loss can stir up in me.

Given that I lost Hannah to suicide, my fear of people dying can understandably take on a life of its own when it comes to a loved one in my life who is deeply struggling emotionally. Volunteer work I've done, my own life experiences, and my field of study have connected me with many people who battle all sorts of addictions, traumas, mental illnesses, etc. I honestly can't count the number of times I've helped talk someone down from suicide or persuaded someone to put down the razor he or she intended to harm him or herself with. I'm humbled and thankful that God can use me to help others, and I know He put this compassion in my heart for people hurting. So it isn't a burden; I love helping people, and I will always be there for anyone who needs support.

Due to losing a close loved one to suicide, though, I've noticed that the nervousness and fear I feel in situations where a friend is suicidal or in a dark place has intensified. I have to be careful, because I know that the pain of wishing I could have stopped Hannah that night will often lead me to overextend and deplete myself in my efforts to save others. I sometimes slip into an irrational mindset of determination to not let anyone else in my life die by suicide.

Realistically, though, that's not possible. I don't have the power to save people. I can't allow myself to feel the pressure of being responsible for the lives of everyone around me. When I succumb to that mentality, I get drained very quickly and it isn't healthy for me. I can't take care of myself if I'm giving everything I have to others. And frankly, I really won't be an effective support for someone if I don't take care of myself as well. So I've been working on maintaining healthy boundaries and knowing my limits. Like the flight attendants always say, we have to put on our own oxygen mask before we help others put on theirs.

Since Hannah's death, I've noticed a significant increase in this fear and it can take me to a place of irrational and paranoid thoughts more often than I like to admit. I still wrestle with it, of course, so I continue trying to work on it. I know that if I let my fears overtake me and consume me, I'll suffocate from the weight of them. And then I would truly be of no help at all to anyone in my life who needs me.

*

CHRISTINE BASTONE
Christine's sister Elizabeth
died in 2012 at age 38

I am most afraid of losing someone else to suicide. Of course I fear losing someone I know and love the most. But this fear includes anyone I know, no matter how casually. This is especially true of people in my online support groups. I consider every fellow member a friend. I consider this to be true whether we are officially friends on Facebook or not, whether we have had any contact with each other or not. It doesn't matter, they are still my friends.

I can handle other people's suicidal thoughts and feelings, especially since I still have these myself. But if I feel someone is actively suicidal, I just about fall apart. I am immediately and automatically in a panic. I don't run into it a whole lot, but I do once in a while. This was especially true when I was an administrator for a number of Facebook groups.

The thoughts are pretty scary when it's your child who is having them! I was shocked speechless when my son mentioned them the first time. And scared when he mentioned them the second time. Thankfully, his school, my son, and I worked together to fix enough of what was bothering him at school, and he's okay now. Fortunately, these feelings didn't last very long.

Sadly, this fear of losing someone to suicide again has already come true once. A Facebook friend of mine died by suicide. We had been friends only for about a year. And it's not like we had a whole lot of interaction, although I did read a number of things that she posted. But it still hit me pretty hard. I considered her a friend, I cared about her, I really liked her, and thought that she was an awesome writer. I was so shocked. And it vividly brought back my initial grief for my sister. It's been a little over a year now, and although I don't grieve for her twenty-four hours a day, it still really

201

hurts. So even though this fear of losing others to suicide has already happened again, I don't fear it any less than I did before.

*

SHARON EHLERS

Sharon's best friend Joy died in 2009 at age 52
Sharon's former fiancé John died in 2012 at age 59

I thought about this question for a long time. Since I wasn't quite sure how to answer, I looked up the definition of "afraid" and saw it has three components: (1) filled with fear or apprehension; (2) filled with concern or regret over an unwanted situation; and (3) having a dislike for something. I couldn't think of anything that makes me afraid as the result of Joy's and John's deaths. I don't feel filled with fear, concern or dislike for something. Okay, I dislike suicide, but I am not afraid.

The only part of the definition that resonated with me was the "regret over an unwanted situation." Since I loved both Joy and John, did I feel regret over their suicides? Of course! I feel sad and sorry for the fact that they both decided to take their own lives. But I worked hard not to make myself feel guilty in anyway. I did at first for Joy. I was the last friend, besides her husband, to talk with her. What did I say or do? What could I have said or done differently?

Eventually I was told that using the word "guilt" implies intent to harm. Never did my actions or lack of action intend to harm Joy in any way. I felt I had nothing to feel guilty about. I tried to help her the best I knew how. Could I have done or said things differently? Of course. Don't most people feel that way? The feeling of wishing you had done things differently is unresolved grief, not guilt. Was it my fault that they both decided to commit suicide? No, it was their decision. A decision I probably couldn't have done anything to change even if I had tried.

So the bigger question is, do I have any other fears associated with their deaths? Am I afraid that someone else I know will try to commit suicide? To be honest, I haven't really even thought about it. After being part of a Survivors After Suicide support group, it became more evident that there wasn't much that anyone who attended could have done to prevent their loved one's death. Not even all the love in the world would have helped. It was out of our hands. It was a personal choice made by the deceased. Many of the participants said they never saw any signs. It was a complete shock to them. One day they were there; the next day they were gone.

So, realistically, do we ever know for sure what is going on in someone's mind? Probably not. If they don't want to help themselves, then there is little we can do. The death of Robin Williams brought suicide to the forefront of mainstream discussions. I think there is increased awareness on this topic. We now know more about the warning signs, but even when you know those things, how much influence can you have on someone who is suicidal? To me it isn't something that I have chosen to worry about.

As a spiritual person, I try to turn any fears and worries I may have over to God, the angels, the universe, etc. Sometimes it is easier said than done, but at least I try. This has helped me not to be fearful nor afraid of the future and things I can't really control. I don't want to spend my life worrying so much about what could happen that I miss living in the present moment. Being afraid and fearful just doesn't work when you are trying to live a full life.

One thing John's death did bring to the forefront, although not really a fear, was making sure you have "everything in order," especially if you are a parent. John chose to leave his mother and his children with a financial and legal mess. They were thrust into a world they never should have had to deal with. There was no will. There was no money. Seeing this made me realize that I needed to make sure everything was in place for my own children. Although

I've had a will since my first daughter was born, I made sure it was up to date and in order. I made sure I had a file with all my important papers, account numbers, insurance papers, etc. I made sure all my children know how to get to it. I think the fear of seeing the impact of John's suicide on his family made me extra diligent not to leave that kind of mess for my own children.

*

BONNIE FORSHEY
Bonnie's son Billy
died in 1993 at age 16

I am afraid of losing another loved one to suicide. It is so abnormal and very hard to cope with. I was afraid of going into that hospital again. But on the first anniversary of Billy's death, I suffered a heart attack and was transported by ambulance to the hospital. I was panicking the entire way, hoping they wouldn't put me in the same room Billy had been in. Well, they did put me in the exact same room that my son had died in, and I really began having problems. I told them what had happened, and they sedated me and moved me into coronary care unit. What are the odds??

*

LAURA HABEDANK
Laura's brother Brian
died in 2010 at age 35

I'm realizing that I'm afraid of spending my golden years alone. I'm divorced, live by myself, and have no children. I always figured that years from now, after my parents had passed on, that Brian and I would have each other to rely on. Now that he's gone I fear that I'll be spending my golden years with absolutely zero family to speak of. I guess it doesn't scare me so much as it just makes me sad.

I have shared this with only a few people until now, but there was a brief period shortly after Brian died when I was considering trying to have a baby with my ex-husband. Those feelings didn't last long, fortunately, because it would have been a terrible idea. I've never had the urge to have children at any point in my life, and the fears of dying alone and of my family's gene pool dying with me were terrible reasons to have reconsidered that, even briefly.

But my deepest fear, by far, is the fear of my own depression. I've struggled with it for as far back as I can remember. I have so many memories of feeling suicidal throughout my entire life, dating back to my early childhood. For the most part I have it under control now, but I'm always afraid of when the next episode is going to hit, because they are absolutely unbearable. I hate the feeling of utter hopelessness and worthlessness that come along with the episodes, and the amount of effort it takes to just get through each day. It's so exhausting—week after week after week. Sometimes the idea of having to go back to the doctor, re-evaluate my prescriptions and adjust the dosage, or the dreaded change of medication altogether, is just so overwhelming. It's hard to muster up the energy to go through all of that—the tapering off of one medication, the ramping up of a new one, and praying the side effects won't be worse than the depression itself and that it will actually work; because if it doesn't, you start the whole difficult process back over again.

*

VICKI HECKROTH
Vicki's son Matthew
died in 2000 at age 17

We argued right before Matt's death about whether he really paid for car insurance or not. They told me he had not, and thus was not covered for his accident. I was very angry, as I believed he was lying to me. I found out six months after his death that he actually had paid the agent but somehow it never got applied. They sent me a refund with an apology. This was part of what pushed him over the edge. We were being sued by the lady Matt hit and ended up having to file bankruptcy.

I am afraid Matt will still be angry with me for not believing him. And that I let him down because I had to file bankruptcy on both his accident and his funeral. It makes me sad thinking about it. I hope I didn't let him down.

*

MARLISE MAGNA
Marlise's fiancé Blaine
died in 2010 at age 36

I can't say I fear anything (besides bugs!). I guess the only real fear I have would be another loss, especially of my parents. Lately I lie awake thinking about this. I'd be utterly lost. I don't fear my own death, though. I just fear not living my life before my end.

*

MARCELLA MALONE
Marcella's brother Michael
died in 2014 at age 20

Since the loss of Michael, I am most afraid of not doing my best to prevent any of my loved ones, or simply those I meet each day, from feeling so helpless that they make the same decision he did. I make sure I am there when anyone needs me, and I am extra conscious of the necessity of ending each conversation with an "I love you," or some other positive departure. The little things are what I am most afraid of missing out on. My outlook on life has definitely changed. This comes out the most when it comes to my parenting. My son just celebrated his first birthday, but my biggest fear is going through the pain my parents live with each day. It's unimaginable and unbearable.

*

JULIE MJELVE

Julie's husband Cameron

died in 2011 at age 42

What I'm most afraid of is this: what if something happens to me? What will then become of my children? We don't have family that is close to us, either geographically or emotionally. They've already lost their father, so now I'm all they have left.

What. If. Something. Happens. To. Me.

*

BRIDGET PARK

Bridget's brother Austin

died in 2008 at age 14

I am afraid that one day my children will ask if I have any siblings and how my brother died. I remember when my mother first told me that her brother had died, and it was very confusing to me. She told me that he got sick and died, but she was just protecting me from the fact that he died by suicide.

I am deathly afraid for this day. If and when it comes, not only does it pain me, but I can relate to my children's curiosity and confusion on the subject. It made me sad as a child to have missed out on having an uncle and possibly having cousins.

I would never tell my children the truth about my brother's death if they ask me when they are too young to understand. I would lie to them as my mother did to me, for their own protection. I do not think it is wrong at all to do so for their own protection.

207

When we tell the stories of our loved one
It not only brings joy to our saddened hearts,
but provides others a brief lesson in
love and loss, gratitude and grace.
DAPHNE GREER

*

CHAPTER SIXTEEN

OUR COMFORT

Life is made up, not of great sacrifices or duties,
but of little things, in which smiles and kindness,
and small obligations given habitually, are what
preserve the heart and secure comfort.
-HUMPHRY DAVY

Transition sometimes feels as if we have embarked on a foreign journey with no companion, compass, or light. Rather than fill our bag with necessities, we often seek to fill it with emotional items that bring us comfort as we find our way through the eye of the storm. What items or rituals bring you the most comfort?

*

KAYLA ARNOLD
Kayla's uncle Tim
died in 2001 at age 34

The things that bring me comfort are sometimes the same things that bring pain: the memories, pictures, the University of Michigan, and football. For me those are things that connect me to my uncle, and things I cherish, but some days they bring me pain and sadness because he is gone. I do find comfort in talking about my uncle, sharing his life and feeling like I kind of still give him a voice. I tend to talk to my mom about my uncle a lot. It is not uncommon at all for her and I to spend time together and bring up random moments, memories or stories about him. Most of the time we end up crying, but that's okay, because those are moments that are so comforting and we can feel him with us. I found comfort in getting a tattoo in memory of my uncle. That was a big part of my grieving process. It helped me and added another level of connection between him and me, and I also use it as a way to keep him around in this world. Many times people ask me who Tim is, and I have the pleasure of telling them he was my uncle. Sometimes they ask how he died, and I am straightforward with them and sometimes I even use the conversation as a way to do some education and prevention.

Overall, I find comfort with my family and our undying love for the most amazing man I have the honor of calling my uncle!

*

EMILY BARNHARDT

Emily's friend and roommate Hannah

died in 2014 at age 20

In looking back, I can pinpoint periods of time where the things that brought me the most comfort altered or became entirely opposite from each other. It's common for our avenues of comfort to change, because WE change. As grief changes us and as we go through the different stages of it, the ways we feel most comforted will also adapt to wherever we are at that point in time. As long as we don't seek comfort in self-destructive or unhealthy behaviors, there's no right or wrong avenue to finding solace in grieving a loss. And those avenues of comfort will vary for each individual.

For example, Hannah's parents had a difficult time looking at pictures of her for a period of time after she passed; it was too painful for them. I, on the other hand, clung to pictures of Hannah and me for dear life and looked at them constantly. Later in my journey, however, there was a period of time when I couldn't handle looking at pictures of Hannah. There was a period of time when I found comfort in looking at or holding Hannah's belongings, and a period of time when I avoided that because it was too hard.

Hannah loved rollerblading, and I always teased her lovingly about it, because hardly anyone rollerblades anymore. She had always tried to get me to go with her, and I'll always regret that I never did. So I knew it would bring me comfort some day to put on her rollerblades and go rollerblading in memory of her. It took a long time before I was ready, but I finally did it one day with a friend who also happened to like rollerblading and came with me for emotional support. We had a good time, and doing it in Hannah's rollerblades made me feel like she was there with me too.

There were seasons throughout my grief when, for various reasons, my main sources of comfort weren't related to Hannah at all. I remember that in the first few months after her death there was a period of three to four weeks where I binge-watched a TV show on Netflix every day. The show had ten seasons, and for those few weeks that show was my life. If I wasn't out at something I was required to be at, then I was lying on my couch at home watching episode after episode. One day I watched it for eight hours straight. It wouldn't have been healthy had it continued for a long time, but for those few weeks it was what I needed, and that's okay.

During the first fall and winter season without Hannah, my avenue of comfort was doing craft projects. This was something I'd never really done before, and it erupted out of nowhere. Searching various do-it-yourself holiday and home décor crafts sites online was a daily activity, and I jokingly tell people that my best friends during that time were my hot glue gun, spray paint, and the crafts store. I made so many craft decorations that I could barely fit them all in my apartment. I felt absolutely insane until a fellow survivor of suicide loss, in order to show me that I wasn't crazy, told me that she herself had made a thousand paper cranes in the first year after her son took his life. We had a good laugh over our absurd crafting. It was good for me, though; it helped me cope at the time. I also found comfort in finishing projects that Hannah and I had previously started and then abandoned, or in following through with ideas we'd had or plans we wanted to do but never did.

The most beautiful gift I gave myself was simply accepting and following that continually changing pathway to comfort wherever it led me, no matter how odd those coping skills might have seemed to me at times. I allowed myself to deal with my grief in whatever way I needed to, as long as it wasn't unhealthy. And I know it was one of the best things I did for myself at that time.

Generally, although there are certain times when I can't handle it, I usually feel most comforted by sentimental things or memories related to Hannah: looking at pictures of us, wearing the necklace she wore almost every day, watching videos of her, reading cards or letters she wrote me, and wearing her clothes. Those things will always be my most precious connection to her, because they allow me to reflect on all the wonderful memories we shared together, the beautiful person she was, and how deeply I will always love and appreciate her for the impact she had on my life.

*

CHRISTINE BASTONE
Christine's sister Elizabeth
died in 2012 at age 38

Anything that makes me feel connected to my sister brings me comfort. This could mean eating something that she liked, seeing the sign from her of "210," feeling her presence, hearing her voice inside my head...anything and everything that makes me feel connected to her. A close second is when anyone mentions her name, or otherwise remembers or honors her. And by "remember," I don't just mean the people who actually knew Liz while she was alive. There are a lot of people in my online support groups who have asked me about her, or made a comment to me about her, or have attended my Facebook event that I have every year for Liz, who have never met her. But when they do those things, it still greatly comforts me. As to the subject of suicide, what brings me the most comfort is anyone who has been suicidal but is still here.

*

SHARON EHLERS
Sharon's best friend Joy died in 2009 at age 52
Sharon's former fiancé John died in 2012 at age 59

After Joy died, what brought me the most comfort was wearing her guardian angel bracelet. I bought it for her as a gift, and after she died her husband agreed I could have it. I wore it all the time. It made me feel like a piece of her was always with me. Eventually it broke. After fixing it twice, the jeweler indicated it couldn't be fixed any more. I was devastated. Maybe it was a sign that it was time to move forward with my grief. Now it sits in my jewelry box. I am content just knowing it is there.

After John died it was a little tougher. We had broken up, so I didn't have a lot of his personal possessions around. Household possessions gave me a piece of him, but it just wasn't the same as having something personal. I had jewelry John had given me, but somehow it didn't seem right to wear it. In those first few days I searched for things that were tangible reminders of him. I would even go to the men's cologne aisle so I could smell the cologne he used to wear. I am sure people thought I was crazy. Maybe more important, I began to think that I was crazy for doing that. I just felt desperate for something familiar. There were so many nights I remember laying my head on his chest in bed after he showered and smelling that smell. I wanted to replicate it somehow, but it just wasn't working. I gave up trying.

A short time later I started to smell his cologne when I was out. If someone was with me I would say, "Do you smell that?" Most of the time they would say they didn't. I would stand behind men who I thought might have it on, only to find out it wasn't coming from them. Then I realized it was John's sign to me. This brought me to tears. It meant he was around me. It meant he must have been watching my nose stalking the cologne counter and smelling all those other men. What a laugh he must have had. At least he knew it was important to me. I am guessing this is why, every now and then, that familiar smell still comes out of nowhere. This is still one of the most comforting smells in the world to me.

Talking to other people about both Joy and John also brings great comfort. I don't avoid it. Society has conditioned us not to open up or really talk about those who have died, especially if they died from suicide. So it becomes an avoided conversation. It's like they never existed. I like talking about them. They had lives that mattered. This is what I talk about. I share personal memories and funny stories with people who did or didn't know them. Talking about them brings me peace. I often find that if I am comfortable it helps the other person to open up and talk about them too.

For those who didn't know Joy or John, it often helps them to open up about their own personal loss stories. You can tell they feel relieved, just like I do, when they can actually talk about the people they loved. So many people are just too afraid to ask, or too afraid to listen. Sharing and receiving those stories is something I will always find to be very comforting.

*

BONNIE FORSHEY
Bonnie's son Billy
died in 1993 at age 16

I love my photos of my son; they are all I have left of his life. I am at peace now. I am comforted by my bittersweet memories, music, and photos. I have two grandsons who look and act like Billy. They bring me so much happiness and help me to cope.

*

LAURA HABEDANK
Laura's brother Brian
died in 2010 at age 35

For me, it is so comforting to know that Brian isn't suffering anymore. Depression is such a cruel and unforgiving illness. I found out only five months before Brian took his own life that he had attempted suicide twice before, once when we were roommates in our mid-twenties. I had no idea that he and I were both experiencing periods of such darkness at the same time, in rooms ten feet from each other. We lived together, ate together, went to movies together yet neither of us wanted to burden the other with the heaviness we were feeling. As much as I hate to admit this, there was a small part of me that was relieved when he died, because I'd spent the previous months in agony wondering if he was okay and panicking each time he didn't answer his phone. I was relieved that he was now free of the darkness that had been weighing him down his entire life.

It also brings me so much comfort to talk about Brian and reminisce over photographs and emails and mementoes. In the beginning I didn't do much of it, because it was still too hard and the panic attacks were never far behind; I had to know my limits and know when I was in a good place to sit down with those things and just have a good cry. Nowadays I find myself smiling more when going through my pictures of him, and I feel less agony and a little more peace because I think I've done a good job of grieving exactly as I needed to—I never forced myself to ignore the feelings that came up; I felt them, processed them and let them go. After five years of that, I'm in a place where there are more smiles than tears when I talk about him. I've received a great deal of comfort from meeting other survivors, particularly other sibling survivors. Losing someone to suicide complicates the grieving process, I believe. Aside from the intense pain and sadness, there are the added feelings of guilt, shame, anger, shock, abandonment, and even relief, as I mentioned earlier. It can be such an alienating experience, because very few people know what to say, so they end up either saying the wrong things or ignoring the bereaved altogether. I met some wonderful friends, fellow sister survivors, at a suicide loss support group, and have met some amazing people through my occasional volunteer efforts regarding suicide awareness and prevention. I was also fortunate enough to be included in a documentary about sibling suicide produced by Caley Cook, entitled *Four Sisters*. The other three sisters also live here in Austin, Texas, and have become my friends. We don't often see each other, but it's been wonderful to be able to get together and know that we all understand one another in a way that others don't. It was difficult to talk about and even more difficult to see it on film two years later, but there was also some incredible healing that came to me because of it, and it felt good to be in a position to help other people going through the same thing.

A few days after Brian died, a family friend gave us a poem about pennies being little reminders that our loved one is letting us know they are around. I didn't think too much of the poem at first, but when we were going through Brian's things it came to mean so much more. When cleaning out his bedroom, the last thing I emptied was his clothes hamper. After I removed the clothes, I carried all the bags I'd collected out into the living room, leaving the hamper where I had found it. About half an hour later my mom went back in there to get the hamper from his room, and she came out with a such look on her face, a look of awe, hope, and pain all at the same time. She stretched out her hand and showed me something she found when she lifted the hamper from its place. It was a single penny. Thinking back to the poem about the pennies, I felt myself choking up. But it got better. I turned the penny over to see that it was dated 1975, the year Brian was born. I immediately burst into tears, and it made my heart smile to think that Brian sent that penny to let us know he was there. I have been collecting all the pennies I find since he passed. I tend to find them in the strangest places and at moments just when I need them most.

*

VICKI HECKROTH
Vicki's son Matthew
died in 2000 at age 17

Being with my grandkids brings me comfort. Even though only one of the ten knew Matthew, I love telling them about their uncle Matt, making sure they all know him through the memories of me and my daughters. I also draw comfort both from talking to him and through my faith. Knowing I will see him again someday, be able to apologize, and tell him how much I love him.

*

MARLISE MAGNA
Marlise's fiancé Blaine
died in 2010 at age 36

Just after Blaine died I was so afraid of forgetting all our memories, so I obsessively started writing them down. Every now and then I will take it out and read through it and die a thousand little deaths. I also sometimes wear a ring of mine he used to wear. Also, knowing he's at peace now brings me comfort.

*

MARCELLA MALONE
Marcella's brother Michael
died in 2014 at age 20

I find the most comfort in the simple things that remind me of Michael. My favorite thing is his Red Wings windbreaker. He got it at a game we went to a year prior to his death. It's one of my many fond memories with him. If I'm having a particularly rough day, I'll put it on to remind myself that I have the best angel looking out for me, making sure I will make it through the challenges life throws my way. Wearing it is like getting a hug from Michael, reminding me he is still there whether I see him or not.

*

JULIE MJELVE
Julie's husband Cameron
died in 2011 at age 42

The thing that brings me the most comfort is to acknowledge that I hurt, that I grieve, that I am sad. Trying to hide all those emotions just makes it hurt worse. I feel better when I don't have to hide it. I made myself a few different variations of a mourning symbol to wear. It started out with a black craft ribbon wrapped around my wedding band. I ended up wearing it for a year, it became a kind of ritual. After that year, I was able to get a silicone bracelet with mourning symbols on it, and I wore that for about another year.

It's hard to find the words to describe how they bring me comfort, but they really do. Somehow they allow me to express those deep emotions that I can't find words for. They make me feel like I've stopped hiding, and have acknowledged the pain I'm in. That's what brings me comfort.

CHAPTER SEVENTEEN

OUR SILVER LINING

Even a small star shines in darkness.
-FINNISH PROVERB

In the earliest days following loss by suicide, the thought that anything good can come from our experience is beyond comprehension. Yet some say there are blessings in everything. Whether one's loss reveals the kindness of a stranger or becomes the fuel to unfurl a new leaf, each silver lining, no matter how small, yields a light in the darkness. Have you discovered a silver lining in your loss?

*

KAYLA ARNOLD
Kayla's uncle Tim
died in 2001 at age 34

The silver lining in the loss of my uncle is being able to help others by spreading education of what to look for in a suicidal friend or loved one, and being able to be a support system for someone who has also lost a loved one to suicide. We are a group of people unlike anyone else. Survivors of loved ones lost by suicide have an undeniable understanding of what others are going through. We know their pain, heartache, and suffering.

We understand how hard it is to get out of bed, how hard it is to try to move on knowing that someone you loved chose to leave you. And we know what it is like to have to live with the fact that we might never know why our loved one is really gone, what his real reason for leaving was, or why he would ever do what he did.

Suicide is the hardest death to deal with because it is a death with no answers. You don't have a definite disease that indicates this is why your loved one is not here. We don't have some random accident as a cause. We have no answers, and we get to spend the rest of our lives wondering *why*?!

Being able to be a support system and an advocate for suicide prevention is one of my biggest silver linings. I am thankful that I view this as an opportunity to save lives and to be a support for those who know my pain, because it makes me feel like my uncle didn't die for nothing, that even though he is not with me I am keeping his memory alive and I am doing my best to help others not have to feel the pain and suffering my family and I have. I am able to help others who are feeling the pain I feel, and we are able to be there for one another. I would love to have my uncle here and not need to have this in common with others, but at the same time it has given me a purpose. It has given me a reason and a way to help others, and it has allowed me to slowly heal my own wounds.

*

EMILY BARNHARDT
Emily's friend and roommate Hannah
died in 2014 at age 20

For the first year after Hannah's death, I wasn't even able to fathom the idea that any sort of future blessing could come out of such a tragic and devastating loss. It felt wrong to even think of calling anything coming as a result of her death a blessing. To me, it felt like I would be saying that her dying was okay. But as I've grown in the journey, I've learned to see it differently. Before, I couldn't connect death with blessing. Now, I'm experiencing how they can indeed coexist. Death and blessing can have a correlative relationship. Many great, courageous and life-changing efforts from people are born out of their experiencing some great sorrow or hardship. Both sorrow and suffering expand the capacity of our hearts to love, to empathize and to show compassion. Sorrow instills a delicate and unique frequency in our hearts that allows us to tune in to that same frequency that weakly exudes from the hearts of others who are hurting. It's a frequency that can often only be heard by those who've heard it personally themselves. The depth of empathy and tenderness we gain in our sorrow allows us a greater capacity to bleed alongside other bleeding hearts, to cry tears for another's pain, and to offer a tight and safe grip for someone to grab onto and trust. It's something that can't simply be taught; it's a beautiful gift that can arise only from the dark debris of despair.

I have believed for most of my life that God has given me a passion and heart for the hurting. The times I feel most blessed are the times when I'm able to help another. And I know that God has used the pain of losing Hannah to deepen, mature, and ignite this part of me. The fire inside my heart to help others, to be an advocate for those suffering, to bring light to those who think they're in darkness too deep to reach, to be a voice, is brighter than it's ever been. It's honestly so bright that it's overwhelming at times! But it's a good overwhelming. It's the brightness of purpose, meaning, passion and hope.

I've grown in many areas of my life because of having to walk through the grief of losing Hannah. I'm continually learning to be a better friend to those hurting. I'm learning more and more the power and intention of the words I say and the way I offer support to others. In my grief, I've experienced God and His character in a way I never did before. I've seen an entirely new depth to His faithfulness, compassion, patience and gentleness. I've also learned the value of true friendship and community. I've witnessed the beauty in relationships that can weather even the fiercest of storms.

The most beautiful and concrete silver lining I've seen in losing Hannah is the door that God's has opened for me to write. It's a door I never would have chosen. It's a door I would reject in a heartbeat if I had the chance to have her back. I've always dreamed, though, that my love of writing could someday make a difference and impact others somehow. Until now, my true writing has been seen only by the "Documents" folder on my laptop and by a few close friends. So I hope to use this opportunity to be an advocate in the things that matter to me, to be a voice and light in the darkness, and to speak words of hope that will transfer into the hearts of people who read or hear them. I know that not everyone who reads my words will share my Christian beliefs when I mention them, and that's okay, because I'm not addressing my words only to a Christian audience. I'm addressing my words to those of you who are grieving the loss of a suicide, and my hope is that something I say can bring you a feeling of comfort, hope, encouragement, or even just the precious feeling of not being alone in your pain.

Hannah's death was not a good thing. It never will be. I will always love her and miss her. I will always be sad that her life ended that way and that soon. I can't change what happened. I can't go back and change it. What I can do, however, is choose what I'm going to do with it. Only I can decide how I will let it change me. I can't take away the pain of losing Hannah, but I can determine to take that pain and do something good with it. And I know for a fact that it's what Hannah would want. She would want her story to help others. This very second, I can hear her voice, the many times and situations when she encouraged me to pursue my dreams and take hold of the opportunities in front of me. Two years ago I was asked to share my story of the things I've walked through in life in front of around thirty people. I was terrified and hesitant, but

Hannah passionately encouraged me, telling me that I would make a difference and help so many people with my story. Hannah believed in me and my potential. So I know the best gift I can give her and her memory is to use her story to help people and make a difference as well.

*

CHRISTINE BASTONE
Christine's sister Elizabeth
died in 2012 at age 38

I am very motivated to not die by suicide myself. I have also learned quite a bit, such as how to help myself when I'm suicidal, how it feels to lose a loved one to suicide, how casually our society throws around all the words connected to suicide like "kill myself" and "hang in there," how often the subject of suicide is seen as funny in sitcoms and comedies, how important it is to remove the stigma and the shame for seeking help, and also how important it is to speak up and not be silent about suicide.

*

SHARON EHLERS
Sharon's best friend Joy died in 2009 at age 52
Sharon's former fiancé John died in 2012 at age 59

I am fortunate that I have been given two silver linings. My first silver lining is knowing that love can get you through just about anything, even heartbreak. It would have been easy to let the grief resulting from Joy's and John's suicides send me into a world of despair. I could have allowed these circumstances to also make me a victim. I could have swaddled myself up in the pain and stopped living my own life. But Joy and John would never have wanted that for me. If they wouldn't have wanted it for me, why would I want it for myself? I am just grateful for their love.

Joy taught me true friendship. She taught me that friends support each other no matter what. John taught me to love from the depths of my soul. He taught me that love knows no boundaries. I know that Joy and John are always with me, cheering me on and offering me comfort when I need it most. I know Joy is working with the angels on a daily basis. I know John is watching over me and my children to keep us safe. I feel their love in everything I do. So the reality is, love doesn't end when someone dies. It continues. Their love made me a better person. There is a quote from Paulo Coelho, author of *The Alchemist* (one of my favorite books), "When we love, we always strive to become better than we are. When we strive to become better than we are, everything around us becomes better too." My life is better because of the love I shared with Joy and John. What better silver lining could there be?

My second silver lining has been taking my grief and finding a way to help others who are grieving. I have to admit that Joy's and John's suicides sent me into a tailspin. But they also made me re-evaluate what is important in life. My children. My family. My friends. Being happy. Living in the present moment.

Their deaths made me think about what really wasn't working for me anymore. As a result, my career jumped to the front of the line. Sure, I had done very well for almost thirty years. I just didn't feel fulfilled anymore. Maybe it was too many years doing the same thing and seeing that nothing was really changing. Was I making great money? Yes. But it wasn't about the money. It was about doing something meaningful. Something that made me happy. My grief journey helped me to recognize this, and I started to look for new adventures. I became a master in the Japanese healing art of Reiki. I also became a Certified Grief Recovery Specialist so I could help others on their own grief journeys. In 2014 I started my own business, Grief Reiki, to provide a multidimensional approach to grief and loss by offering emotional recovery and spiritual healing. Now there are infinite possibilities of where life can take me. For me, this has brought a silver lining to what started as a cloudy and stormy period in my life.

*

BONNIE FORSHEY
Bonnie's son Billy
died in 1993 at age 16

There is no silver lining in suicide, not for me. I lost my son and I lost myself. It destroyed our lives and forever changed my daughter. My son's suicide led to the suicide of one of his friends. I have gone on to speak with other teens who have attempted suicide, and after telling them my story they have been able to turn their lives around. They have gone through counseling and are leading happy lives. So I guess there is a silver lining for them, but not for me.

*

LAURA HABEDANK
Laura's brother Brian
died in 2010 at age 35

It could be the suicide loss, and it could just be my getting older and more mature, or a combination of both, but I've grown stronger. I can handle more than I ever dreamed possible. I am getting better at sticking up for myself more, and I find that I'm more likely to rid myself of relationships that are harmful to me or don't serve me well. Throughout a number of difficult losses in my life since Brian died, I've reminded myself that I will get through it. If I can manage to survive losing Brian like I did, I can surely overcome other losses too. I've become more open with others about my own struggle with depression, self-injury, and suicidality. I want to increase awareness for the good of all who suffer from it, but also to help others who have lost someone close to them to suicide. I think I have a unique perspective to offer. Not only have I had someone close to me die by suicide, but I've also been seconds away from taking my own life on multiple occasions. I can understand the mindset behind someone making that choice for himself, as well as the thought process of someone trying to cope with the aftermath of that choice.

This grief journey has also made me more caring toward others. I think anyone who has suffered naturally develops a more compassionate nature, because he knows pain and doesn't wish to see anyone suffer as he has. There are some seemingly benign changes of which I'm aware, like how I relate to others. If I am stuck behind someone at a stoplight who is not moving when the light turns green, my initial reaction is to honk and get him moving again. But then I recall the days and weeks and months following Brian's death when I drove around in a complete daze and would often just space out at a light until I was startled out of my tearful moment of remembrance by the honk of the car behind me. If someone is rude or abrasive toward me, my knee-jerk reaction is to be upset or snap back. But if I take another moment to think about it, I remember how early on I was in a constant state of "fight or flight," and with my emotions so close to the surface I could blurt out things I didn't mean, because I was acting out of pain. I've been trying to remain mindful of the fact that each person is fighting his own kind of battle and to be respectful of that. It's not always easy to do, but I try to be aware of that as much as possible.

Finally, I think this process has helped me become less anxious. Anxiety is still an issue for me, but not to the degree that it used to be. I guess when compared to the death of my brother few things really compare in their importance, and I'm getting better at not obsessing over things that just don't matter. I'm learning how to "pick my battles" within my relationships and try to really focus on the larger issues that are most important to me.

*

VICKI HECKROTH
Vicki's son Matthew
died in 2000 at age 17

My daughters and I have become much closer. My granddaughter Breanna has her Matt story published in a book called, *Heaven Talks to Children*. My grandsons remind me of Matt every day by the way they look and act. My husband and I are much closer, and my husband quit drinking. I have been able to help others who are suicidal or have lost someone to suicide so no other family has to go through this. I give talks, telling my story for schools and institutions. I keep Matt alive in my heart and soul through my speeches.

*

MARLISE MAGNA
Marlise's fiancé Blaine
died in 2010 at age 36

All I can think of as a silver lining is that Blaine is at peace now and it just wasn't meant to be. Also, the fact that it has made me a much stronger person and I found my faith and calling in the process.

*

MARCELLA MALONE
Marcella's brother Michael
died in 2014 at age 20

April 14, 2014, thus far the worst day of my life, the day I had to face the reality that my brother chose to leave this earth and his family behind, has somehow amazingly but slowly shown a silver lining in my life. Don't get me wrong, each day is a struggle and still brings me pain, but my brother's loss has also taught me the value of each day. I had always taken each day for granted, as well as Michael's presence in all the events of my future. After his loss I struggled with the fact that I didn't see it coming and couldn't stop it. I went to my comfort of research and read everything I could find on suicide and sibling loss. I discovered that he was in the highest risk group as a young male. Those seen as the strongest frequently lose their battle with their inside demons. This hit me hard. I began looking at each day as an opportunity to bring a smile to someone's face. I began making time for family and friends. I put in a stronger effort to get along with the other half of my son's family. These people and things are no longer taken for granted. No matter how angry I may be, I do my best to end everything with "I love you." It may not seem like much, but this new outlook on life has made a major impact on my life and greatly assisted in my grief journey.

*

JULIE MJELVE
Julie's husband Cameron
died in 2011 at age 42

Some of the silver lining I was able to recognize right away. With my husband's mental illness, our life together was very difficult. As his life ended, I was able to recognize that he had been set free, that he would no longer be in pain.

It took probably at least a year to be able to see the rest of the silver lining. I have become a stronger person. I'm better able to stand up for myself. I'm better at deciding what I want, what I will accept from others, and better able to communicate those desires. I've become better at handling the stress and anxiety of everyday life. Instead of trying to avoid these situations, I've learned how to work through them, which actually alleviates the stress much more effectively than my previous avoidance tactics.

*

GRACE YOUNG
Grace's son Jack died
in 2007 on his 27th birthday

Our silver lining comes in the form of a day dedicated to helping others. Our family created Particle Accelerator, in Memory of Jack Young Jr., an annual music festival that brings families together to learn about the signs of depression and suicide. It is an informal, fun day that includes local music, our local mental health organization, United Services, Inc., and our Wall of Angels, a photo memorial to those lost to suicide. We know that our day of music and hope saves lives. We have raised over forty thousand dollars in the last eight years for United Services, which uses the funds to teach mental health first aid training to help people recognize the signs of someone having a mental health crisis.

Jack's friends came to us after his death and said they wanted to do something in his honor to educate the public about depression, because they too had not recognized that Jack was suicidal. We make it a fun day for families with balloons, moon bounces, a BMX bike demonstration, a raffle with gifts from local businesses, food, and local vendors. We have a Book Corner that highlights authors and books that can help one cope with depression and grief, a Faith Corner to lead people to God in response to depression and grief, an Art Corner to show that the arts can help ease depression, a Kids Corner to keep kids entertained while their parents listen to the music.

Our Wall of Angels currently has over two hundred dear souls on it from all over the world. It helps people to see how varied the individuals who die by suicide really are: men, women, children, rich, poor, etc. We also have people from the Department of Veterans Affairs join us to teach about suicide in the military, our local drug and alcohol resistance group, called PRIDE, to teach about the dangers of substance abuse when one is depressed, and United Services hands out information about treatment available to help those who are struggling. United Services has seen a huge increase in its caseload as a result of Particle Accelerator, and we are honored to recommend them to those who need help. It has also helped our family come to terms with our devastating loss, knowing that lives that would otherwise be lost can be found again with help.

*

CHAPTER EIGHTEEN

OUR HOPE

*One smile can change a day. One hug can change
a life. One hope can change a destiny.*
-LYNDA CHELDELIN FELL

Hope is the fuel that propels us forward, urges us to get out of bed
each morning. It is the promise that tomorrow will be better than
today. Each breath we take and each footprint we leave is a measure
of hope. So is hope possible in the aftermath of suicide? If so, where
do we find it?

*

EMILY BARNHARDT
Emily's friend and roommate Hannah
died in 2014 at age 20

In every facet of my life, and especially in my grief, I find hope
in Christ. The only time my hope is grounded is when it's in Him –
who He is, what He's done for me, and in His promises. Through
the prior hardships I experienced before Hannah's death, I have
learned just how fully God can heal and restore even the most
shattered pieces of my heart. I've seen how He used those painful
experiences to help and bring hope to others. My witnessing of this
has given me the assurance that He's good, and that there is a

purpose and plan for my life. Without Him, I'm lost. So when I look at this loss through that perspective, I know there is hope for my life. I don't know exactly what it will look like or how it will manifest, but if my hope is in Him, then I will always have hope and confidence in His plan.

I also define hope in helping others. I use the word "define" because it's a verb, and I find hope in the action of helping others and seeing that same hope come into their eyes. I also feel hope whenever I share words of hope. Sometimes, the words I say while trying to give someone else hope are the same words I might need to hear at any given moment. Whenever we speak words of hope, that hope will transfer back to us as well. I find hope when I tell the bereaved that they are courageous for getting out of bed that day. I feel hope and validation when I tell someone that their pain matters, and that it's normal to feel what he is feeling. I also reassure him that he isn't crazy, and nothing is hopeless. I find hope when I encourage someone to show self compassion and patience as he moves through his own grief. I feel hope when I validate the small, daily victories someone else has made. Through my own tears, I find hope when I tell someone that it is okay to cry.

First and foremost, I find hope in God: in His plan, His purpose, and His promises. I then try to cultivate hope for others by making a difference, and try to lift some of the weight off another's back and help them carry it, if even for just a moment. We aren't meant to walk alone. I have hope in our ability to embrace one another in our darkest of nights. And I believe in the hope that comes from it.

*

CHRISTINE BASTONE
Christine's sister Elizabeth
died in 2012 at age 38

Hope is when you believe that some how, some way, things will get better some day. Hope is also the knowledge that one day can change everything. It can be for the worse or for the better. When I lost my sister, of course it was for the worse. I have hope that one day things will change for the better. I feel that hope is also wanting to see how everything turns out. It is living out the saying "Where there is life, there's hope." And not wanting to exit, so to speak, right before things get better!

*

SHARON EHLERS
Sharon's best friend Joy died in 2009 at age 52
Sharon's former fiancé John died in 2012 at age 59

Hope means so many things to me. Hope is seeing life through the eyes of your children. Hope is watching a sunset and knowing you made it through another day. Hope is knowing that if you got through one day, you will get through another. Hope is feeling what it is like to love. Hope is helping others get through tough times. Hope is being a shoulder to cry on. Hope is watching children play at a park. Hope is having a really good cup of coffee. Hope is a rainbow. Hope is walking barefoot in the sand. Hope is seeing a sky full of stars. Hope is watching the seasons change. Hope is watching dreams become a reality. Hope is listening to beautiful music. Hope is getting signs from your loved ones. Hope is recognizing synchronicities. Hope is feeling your loved ones next to you. Hope is believing in a better tomorrow. Hope is having a better tomorrow. Hope is feeling your heart begin to heal. When we finally emerge from tragedy, it is amazing how much hope we can find around us. I have been very blessed to see it every day.

Two of my favorite quotes about hope are:

Hope is being able to see that there is light
despite all the darkness.
BISHOP DESMOND TUTU

Hope is important because it can make the present moment
less difficult to bear. If we believe that tomorrow will
be better, we can bear a hardship today.
THICH NHAT HANH

*

BONNIE FORSHEY
Bonnie's son Billy
died in 1993 at age 16

I would like to see more schools discuss suicide and offer help to any children who might need it. The parents should be notified promptly, so they can get their child the help he or she needs. No one informed me that my son was depressed. He hid it from me, but did tell a friend of his. The parents even found a will that he had written, but never told me. If they had told me, he might still be here.

*

LAURA HABEDANK
Laura's brother Brian
died in 2010 at age 35

I think this is the most difficult of all of these questions for me. I mean, I know what the textbook definition of hope is, but truthfully I just haven't felt a whole lot of it since Brian took his life. I've been capable of feeling happiness and joy and enjoyment, and have been able to laugh again, but so far hope has eluded me. I keep telling myself that the best I can do is to keep moving forward and maybe someday a little hope will come back to my life. I guess you could say that I'm hopeful that one day I'll have hope again. In the words of Forrest Gump, "And that's all I have to say about that."

*

VICKI HECKROTH
Vicki's son Matthew
died in 2000 at age 17

Hope means that one day I will be with my son in heaven again. Each day I get through is one more day with my loved ones here, and one day closer to being with my son again. My hope in God means that all things are possible. My religious beliefs have become very strong. I talk to my son through God, something that everyone should do. Hope is helping others who are depressed; hope is that no other family has to go through this horrific pain.

*

MARLISE MAGNA
Marlise's fiancé Blaine
died in 2010 at age 36

The bible states there is *always* hope, faith and love. Hope to me means things can only get better and that this too shall pass.

*

JULIE MJELVE
Julie's husband Cameron
died in 2011 at age 42

My definition of hope lies in the future. My life, and who I am is not defined by any one single act in the past or the present. Hope, for me, is that there is always a chance for change or for something amazing to happen. I look at the smiles on my children's faces and know there is a future, a future filled with hope.

*

GRACE YOUNG
Grace's son Jack died
in 2007 on his 27th birthday

Hope can raise you up when your heart is heavy, and hope is a powerful thing. We try our best to be hopeful and helpful to our family and friends, and we think our community also benefits from this hope. We have gained strength from hope where once we were lost, and without hope we falter.

*

CHAPTER NINETEEN

OUR JOURNEY

Be soft. Do not let the world make you hard. Do not let the pain make you hate. Do not let bitterness steal your sweetness. -KURT VONNEGUT

Every journey through loss is as unique as one's fingerprint, for we experience different beliefs, different desires, different needs, different tolerances, and often we walk different roads. Though we may not see anyone else on the path, we are never truly alone for more walk behind, beside, and in front of us. In this chapter lies the participants' answers to the final question posed: What would you like the world to know about your grief journey?

*

KAYLA ARNOLD
Kayla's uncle Tim
died in 2001 at age 34

My journey started at a young age, an age when I had no understanding what pain and grief I would go through. I was at an age when I didn't have the slightest idea what suicide was or why someone I loved would even dare to do it. It's been fourteen years of learning, coping, grieving, and healing. Some days it feels like yesterday, but other days it feels like an eternity ago.

As much as it hurts to lose your loved one, don't let his or her death go without a greater purpose. Become an advocate for suicide prevention. Educate people, and be a helping hand for those who are going through the same thing you are. Trust me, it is helpful!

Take part in an Out of Darkness walk near you and raise money for the American Foundation for Suicide Prevention. Make something good come out of the worst thing that ever happened to you. Remember that in most cases there is nothing you could have done to stop the suicide. Don't blame yourself; it only hurts you! Take the time to allow yourself to heal, but also remember that even though your loved one left you before you were ready, know that he loves you, and I am sure he misses you just as much as you miss him. Remember, it never really gets better; it starts getting easier because you just learn to adapt and you learn how to live without him. It is never easy learning how to move on without your loved one here, but if you never do it, you are the one who suffers and the one who lives with the pain. It is easier to allow yourself to heal, smile, laugh, remember, and most important, keep living! I know we have a pain thrown at us that seems unbearable, but in time it gets lighter and we are able to live our lives. Our loved ones would want us to keep living, experiencing, growing, and making new memories. Most important, always remember they are with us!

*

EMILY BARNHARDT
Emily's friend and roommate Hannah
died in 2014 at age 20

The most important thing to know about my journey is that it isn't always uphill. Grieving isn't a linear climb where the various stages of it are completed and checked off one by one. It doesn't work that way. Grief isn't an outline with corresponding deadlines that must be followed; it's an ambiguous experience that must be felt. We aren't in the driver's seat when it comes to experiencing the emotions of grief. We don't get to plug in our destination and choose our route; we have to simply sit in the passenger seat and process the emotions we experience at every turn.

One might read some of the words I've written throughout this book and believe that I have it all down pat, but that isn't true in the slightest. I've found healing and growth in many areas and I've learned a lot of truths about grief, and I want to share those truths with others. I also want readers to know I have days where I feel the exact opposite of something I voiced in this book. It simply demonstrates how grief can often be confusing, upside down, backwards, and exhausting.

For example, I know deep down that I'm not responsible for the events of Hannah's suicide. But sometimes, on particularly fragile and emotional days, I truly believe that I am. I know the blessings and silver linings I've seen God bring out of this devastating loss, but there are also days when I don't see it at all. I try to celebrate my little victories, because I know they're important and they matter, yet there are some days when I beat myself up over the areas I feel I'm falling short in. It's a rollercoaster; the kind that takes unexpected turns and jolts, and just when you think it's about to level out, you suddenly plummet. That's just how grief is, unfortunately. We don't get to build or choose the tracks of the rollercoaster, but we do have to ride it.

I want to use these final words to also address two specific and important issues that often surface while processing this type of loss: anger and self-blame. An honest truth is that many survivors of suicide struggle with feeling angry toward their loved one who died. When a loved one is murdered, the survivors process the anger toward the person who killed him. In loss by suicide, complex grief often results from the reality that the victim and perpetrator are one and the same.

I had moments of feeling very angry at Hannah; I still feel a twinge of guilt and pain even as I write these words. How can I feel angry at someone I love so much, and who was hurting so deeply? That's honestly one of the many reasons why grieving a loss by suicide is its own unique hell: there are contradicting thoughts and emotions involved. There were honestly moments when I wanted to hate Hannah for taking her life. Immediately I would then hate myself for even thinking that, because I knew I could never hate her; I loved her too much. When I dug deeper, I realized that my anger wasn't hateful anger; it was heartbroken anger. It was an anger stemming from love; it stemmed from a place deep within me, where the pain of losing her was so devastating and overwhelming that my desperate mind needed to find a definitive cause and/or someone to blame. And though it was heartbreaking to feel angry at her, I did at times. I was angry at her for giving up and acting so impulsively that night. I was angry at her for leaving me to deal with the pieces of her life and the life we had together, our once intertwined routines were now just fragmented pieces.

I was angry at her for not giving me the chance to help her get through that night. I was angry at her for not calling me, when I made her promise that she'd call if she felt like she was going to do something irrational before I could get to her. I was angry at Hannah for not thinking about what taking her life would do to those who love her. I was angry at her for causing the depth of pain and heartache I felt. I was angry at her, ultimately, because I loved her…and that's why it hurt so deeply.

I also realized that some of that anger I felt wasn't toward Hannah, but rather toward myself. I was angry at myself for the events of that night. Why did I let her hang up the phone? Why didn't I force her to talk to me until I got to her location? I was angry at myself for not seeing the severity of the situation. I was angry that, while out looking for her, I unknowingly drove past her location, the very location where she took her life. So I was angry at myself for not looking harder. I'll always wonder if I could have saved her in that moment, if only I had looked more.

I was angry at myself in general. I berated myself for not loving her better and not helping her more. I was angry at myself for waiting until we met to say what I wanted to say. I was angry at myself for not telling her often enough how much I loved her, cared about her, and what a difference she made in my life.

I was just angry in general and I felt like I failed her. I still have many days when I feel like I failed her. I was angry for a while, because it didn't make sense. And no matter how hard I tried, no matter how deeply I searched within, no matter how much I tormented myself with retracing the events of that night, I still couldn't find any sense to it.

Hannah was an amazing, lively, loyal, driven, passionate, funny, outgoing, and loving girl. She had so much going for her. She had dreams and career goals: to be a nurse, a mother, to get married and to experience life. She worked so hard and never gave up. So it didn't make sense to me. And it didn't seem fair. It still doesn't make sense to me, and I've had to come to terms with the reality that it possibly never will. I could easily spend the rest of my life obsessing over the "what ifs" and all the unanswered questions. But I know that it tortures me when I stay in that place, and Hannah wouldn't want that.

I just want to speak to any of you who currently wrestle with anger, self-blame or the "what-ifs." I want to tell you the same words I've told myself: It's okay to feel whatever you're feeling, even if it's deep anger at your loved one who passed.

You need to allow yourself to ride the waves of emotions as they come and not judge them. You need to have compassion toward yourself. You need to know that your loved one's decision to take his or her life was his or her decision alone. We are never responsible or equipped to keep someone else alive, especially when that person doesn't want to be. When it comes to feelings of guilt or self-blame, I want to remind you that in everyday life we face countless decisions, whether significant or menial. As we go about each day, we're always making decisions. And we'll honestly never know what different choices, even in the menial decisions, might have influenced a different outcome in a situation. We all do the best we can with the knowledge we have in any given moment. That's all we can do.

Sadly, hindsight can often make us feel like we failed though; it will berate us for what we did or didn't do, and tell us that what we did wasn't good enough. Hindsight is cruel in that sense; it creates a false notion that it's possible to live and act perfectly.

In the loss of our loved ones, we have to compassionately accept that we did the best we could with the knowledge we had, which can also mean no knowledge at all. We will drive ourselves crazy with the guilt and "what-ifs." It's our mind's way of trying to make sense of and find answers to something we will never be able to fully understand.

If your loved one told you they were about to take his or her life, you would have done anything to stop them. But they didn't. They didn't tell us their plan, and when and where it would happen. I hope you can find comfort in knowing how deeply you love the person you lost – how you know you would have done everything in your power to save them if you could have. But because your loved one didn't tell you his or her plan, when and where it would happen, that guilt isn't yours to carry.

Our loved ones made a life-altering and heartbreaking decision that they didn't consult us on, so we can't hold ourselves responsible for that. We can't blame ourselves for a decision made without our knowledge, because we know we would've chosen differently for them. And because they made such a devastating decision without us, it's also normal for it to feel like a rejection or an abandonment at times. Just know that you will have an endless range of different emotions, and understand that is common and expected. I believe that the reason we often feel guilty and blame ourselves ISN'T because we realistically should have done or said more, or known what he or she was going to do. I believe that our tendency to feel guilt and to blame ourselves only speaks to the depth of love we have for our loved one, and how desperately we want to find the answers and understand how this happened. Unfortunately, blaming ourselves can falsely feel like a concrete explanation we can grasp when, in reality, we're truthfully just searching for an explanation that can never be concretely defined. We want to understand because we hope that understanding will help us in processing our loss. Search if you need to, just don't let your need to understand project any blame onto you - it's not yours to carry. What you must focus on carrying right now is your grief, your memories, your love for the one you lost, and your fragile heart. Take care of it. Take care of you.

I hope you know that your deep sorrow is a reflection of the deep love you have in your heart. Your sorrow is beautiful evidence of that love, and your grief journey will take as long as it takes. So keep taking steps, no matter how small, and congratulate yourself for the little victories, no matter how insignificant they may seem. Rest when you need to, and take all the time that you need.

*

CHRISTINE BASTONE
Christine's sister Elizabeth
died in 2012 at age 38

What I would like the world to know is that the world looks different after you lose a loved one to suicide. We look at the world through very different eyes. Things that we used to not even notice now hurt more than you can imagine. Many things mean something completely different now. Saying things like "Hang in there," "That blew me away," "I'm dying to…." or "That kills me," or "I'd rather die than…." can upset survivors very much. We wince when we hear joking or casual references to blowing one's brains out, or jumping off a bridge. Not to mention that we find pointing your finger at your head and pretending to shoot yourself downright offensive. Even songs have a different meaning, especially ones like "What doesn't kill you makes you stronger."

Suicide is not funny…ever. People dying tragically is just not funny. I don't know why the subject is on sitcoms so much, but I have to leave the room when it is. More and more I dislike the way the subject is treated on TV. And I don't care that it's just a sitcom or whatever, the subject of suicide should be treated more sensitively. And when it's not, it demeans suicide survivors, suicidal people, and people who have died by suicide. The subject of suicide should never be treated casually or lightly, but always be treated seriously and with respect.

Most people who die by suicide are not selfish. It is extremely common for them to believe that their loved ones would be better off without them. That does not sound like selfishness to me. They are not cowards either. In order to die by suicide, you have to find a way to override our most basic instinct…survival. No coward can do that!

Language is very powerful. I never knew how powerful until after I lost my sister. For example, take terms such as "successful suicide," and "failed suicide attempts." What other subject do we talk about where success means someone has died, and failure means someone lived? That makes absolutely no sense.

Then there's the term "committed suicide." That implies a crime. It's a carryover from the days when suicide was a crime. And it needs to be changed. We need to say that someone "died by suicide" instead of "committed suicide."

Grief from death by suicide is more complicated than other deaths. We are more likely to struggle with unanswered questions, such as why it happened. Not that other kinds of death don't have unanswered questions, but they are a special torture for those of us who are suicide loss survivors.

Suicide loss survivors also typically feel more guilt, blame and responsibility for the death of their loved ones than other grievers. The suicide of a loved one creates a feeling of utter helplessness for those of us left behind. In order to maintain a sense of control, we often blame the deaths of our loved ones on actions that we either took or didn't take. Suicide is a different type of death. It is an act that one's own loved one does. And I can tell you from personal experience that this one fact causes untold anguish.

Suicide loss survivors typically struggle more with feelings of rejection and abandonment by their loved one. Not that other grievers can't feel like their loved ones left them. But at least they have the comfort of knowing that he or she didn't leave voluntarily, and that he or she would have stayed if they could.

Suicide can happen to anyone. Given the right circumstances, any one of us can become suicidal. I believe it is a mistake to think that it can never happen to you. No one is completely immune. But at least with ourselves we have control over our actions. What people need to know even more is that it can happen to any family. Any family, even yours. Because suicide knows no boundaries. None whatsoever.

In my opinion, one thing that we need desperately in this world is understanding. Notice that I did not say "love." There is a whole lot of love in this world. Go to any grief support group and you will see the evidence of an abundance of love. Do we need to express it more, and express it better? Yes, but our love is limitless. Unfortunately, there is not nearly enough understanding. And yet we need understanding too. It's a great comfort to be understood. I think a big reason why we go through struggles is so that we can understand others with the same or similar struggles. In my opinion, the people who give the best advice are those who have been there. This is why I agreed to be a part of this book.

*

SHARON EHLERS
Sharon's best friend Joy died in 2009 at age 52
Sharon's former fiancé John died in 2012 at age 59

This is what I learned on my grief journey: Face your grief head-on. I never wanted grief to be part of my life, but it found me nonetheless. Big time. Twice. Once it found me, I had two choices about how I was going to handle it: bottle it up inside and walk around pretending I was okay, or face it head-on and let the emotions flow. Although it was harder to do, I chose the latter. I knew I had to take the journey even though I didn't want to do it. I knew no one else could do it for me. So I did everything I could to confront it. I cried until there were more no tears. I emptied my sorrows until I felt hollow inside. Slowly but surely I found hope again. I don't think I would be the person I am today if I hadn't "forced" myself to grieve.

My advice is, don't avoid grief. Face it head-on. No matter hard it is, it is part of being human. It means you loved someone. It means you loved someone so much your heart broke into a million pieces. It means you are going to be sad. It means you are going to hurt like heck. But it really means you are going to be okay.

Don't let the grief urban legends get to you. For generations, society handed us too many urban legends about grief. None of them are true. None of them work. We have to face grief in new ways. We have to talk about it. We have to feel it. We have to reach out to others for help. If not for ourselves, then for future generations. I don't want my children putting up walls or shutting down when they lose something they love. I don't want them carrying emotional baggage from relationship to relationship because they can't deal with loss. I want my children to be honest about their emotions. I want them to know it is just as normal to be sad as it is to be happy. I want them to know it is healthy to grieve. I want them to know that although it hurts, they will get through it. I want them to understand this, so they can pass it down to their own children. If everyone can do this then eventually grief will no longer be the taboo subject it is today. We will be able to talk about it. We will be able to handle it together.

Find gratitude in the smallest things. In my case, tragedy showed me how much life matters. Every day I write down one thing that makes me grateful. I place it in a "Gratitude Bucket." I decorated my bucket with a sticker that says "Choose Joy." Coincidental? Not really. At the end of this year I plan to pull out each slip of paper and read it aloud. I am grateful for this day. I am grateful for my children. I am grateful for my family. I am grateful to spend time with friends. I am grateful I live near the ocean. I am grateful I found a parking spot at the supermarket. I am grateful for the taste of banana cream pie ice cream. I am grateful for Joy and her friendship. I am grateful for John and his love. I am grateful that their lives touched mine. I am grateful that life has given me so much. I am grateful that today is a new day. These remind me how much life really matters.

"Do what is right for you." This is the most important lesson of all. Grief is your own journey to take. It's on your own time schedule. It's your own long, winding, often bumpy road. It's really important to understand this. Don't listen to what others say about how you should be grieving. If you are not okay, say so. If you are having a bad day, say so. If you are heartbroken, say so. I know some people don't understand why I still grieve for Joy and John. Why I remember and celebrate their birthdays and grief anniversaries. Why I still talk about them. Why I still talk *to* them.

How I can actually still say their names. But I don't care. Joy and John meant a lot to me. I will never get over them. I have resolved any pain I might have had, and now I just remember the importance of each relationship. There are good days and bad days. There are happy memories and sad memories. This is perfectly okay for me. I am where I am right now because I grieved in a way that was right for me.

I am finally at peace. And I know they are too.

*

BONNIE FORSHEY

Bonnie's son Billy

died in 1993 at age 16

I would ask you to educate yourself about the signs of suicide. Get help for your child or loved one, if he or she is depressed. Remove any weapons from your home and lock up your medications.

*

LAURA HABEDANK

Laura's brother Brian

died in 2010 at age 35

If there is one thing I have learned, it is that there is no right or wrong way to grieve the loss of a loved one. Everyone is different, and what worked for me might not work for another. But sooner or later it does need to be dealt with.

I met a woman in the support group one evening who had lost someone close to her to suicide fifteen years earlier, but had never really allowed herself to grieve. She continued to push her feelings aside year after year, and eventually ended up hospitalized after having a nervous breakdown. She shared with us that she wished she had addressed her feelings years earlier.

There's also no set timeline for grief. The five stages of grief outlined by Elisabeth Kübler-Ross (denial, anger, bargaining, depression, and acceptance) can happen in any order, over and over and in combination with one another. I still find myself experiencing all of these stages, sometimes all in a single day, even five years later. I would want people to know that they should never force themselves, or anyone else, to move through grief any faster than what feels natural to them. There is never an appropriate time to tell someone, "You should be over it by now." The thing is, you don't ever get over it. You get through it and you get better at dealing with it, but you never get over it.

Having my brother choose to die left me feeling abandoned. I once asked him, knowing full well how deeply he was suffering, to promise me he wouldn't leave me. He told me he couldn't promise that. In hindsight, I regret asking that of him, because I know that had that same question been posed to me in the middle of a suicidal episode, I'd have been unable to promise it myself and would have resented anyone who asked it of me. But having been left behind like this, I've become increasingly afraid of abandonment and am working on that as it has certainly complicated some of my relationships and, sadly, even ended a few. I began going to support group meetings for suicide survivors only two weeks after Brian's death, not only because I really needed to talk openly about it, but also because all of my family and closest friends were 1,200 miles away. I desperately wanted to be around others who understood what I was going through. It was so important for me to find a support group specific to suicide, because I don't think I could have been nearly as open about my feelings about my brother's choice to end his own life while surrounded by people who were grieving the losses of people who fought valiant battles against cancer or were tragically killed in an accident. Death is death, but there was something so valuable to be shared among a group of survivors who had to deal with the fact that their loved ones chose to die. I'd also like people to know that a little support toward a grieving friend can go a long, long way. Even if you don't have the perfect words to say (because often those words just don't exist), just being there to listen is such an incredible gift.

*

VICKI HECKROTH
Vicki's son Matthew
died in 2000 at age 17

Even though it seems impossible to get through, you can do it. Accept the help from those who have already walked in our shoes until the day comes when you are finally able to help others. It is okay to cry, even to howl like an animal. Whatever it takes to get the pain out. If you have lost a child and you have other surviving children, don't forget to include them in your grief as well. They are hurting too, and they need you just as you need them. Please do not point the blame finger, as it will only come back to haunt you. Keep your family close, but don't smother them. Never give up on hope, because sometimes that's all you have. If you can, reach out for suicide awareness and prevention, as that will help you in the long run. Helping others always seems to make our grief hurt less.

*

MARLISE MAGNA
Marlise's fiancé Blaine
died in 2010 at age 36

I've learned to take things slowly, ten minutes at a time, if I must. Even though at times it feels like there is no hope and your life is over, time does heal. Also, love is everything, and a small smile or act of kindness helps you feel better. Most of all, have no expectations. Hope for the best, expect the worst, and you will end up somewhere in between. "Life goes on."

*

MARCELLA MALONE
Marcella's brother Michael
died in 2014 at age 20

My grief journey since Michael's death has definitely been an emotional rollercoaster. It's given me a new outlook on the world and helped me to better read the unspoken emotions of those around me. It's given me a new understanding on what I'm learning as I finish up my psychology degree, and, most importantly it has taught me a couple of important lessons. The biggest thing I learned, and am still learning, is to not be afraid to talk about things. It is very unhealthy to hold your emotions in. Talking about Michael's life helps me keep his memory alive and helps others to understand the depth of our loss. Talking about the impact of how he left this earth and how I'm coping with it has helped me to heal and shown me who is really there for me. Through conversation I have found a support that I could have never found myself through strangers and those close to me. Your journey should not be alone. It also taught me the absolute value of those you love, and every day you are given together. It taught me not to hold grudges and to never miss an opportunity to tell someone how you feel about him or her. Life is way too short.

The biggest lesson it taught me was to never judge a book by its cover. Everyone has struggles, and frequently those who are better at hiding them are suffering a harder battle. It takes only a few seconds to be kind, and it's so worth it. With this positivity, I also want to tell readers that grief takes time. It's been almost nineteen months but it still feels like yesterday. Don't let others' expectations that you should feel fine cause you to suppress your feelings. Your journey is your own. Cry when you need to, talk when you need to, laugh when you need to, and be angry when you need to. It will pass until the next episode occurs. This is the hardest part of grief.

Nobody likes to talk about death, but I'm grateful that this book has given me the opportunity to talk about Michael. As the sibling, I frequently feel like my grief is overshadowed. The pain my brother's death has brought my parents is unimaginable, and as I have become a parent since his loss, I have a stronger sense of that loss. I am there for my parents at every opportunity, and always will be. It feels wrong for me to say that some days I wish people would see the impact the loss of my brother and best friend has had on me. Before becoming a parent, outliving him was always my bigger fear. I still can't imagine the big events of my future without him. Every day I'm asked about how my parents are since his death, but no one has asked me since the funeral. I answer their questions with a smile on my face, but it has given me the incentive to always check on the siblings after a loss, and let them know I'm thinking of them. I know it would mean the world if someone did the same for me. To whoever is reading this, your pain and your journey matter. I may not know you, but I love you, and I am always thinking and praying for you.

*

JULIE MJELVE
Julie's husband Cameron
died in 2011 at age 42

I would like the world to know first and foremost that grief is indeed a journey. It is not a one-time event, it is something I will carry with me for the rest of my life. While it will move from the foreground to the background, it will still be there. It's not something I will "get over," and most certainly not in two or three weeks. I would like the world to know that the initial intense grief lasts more like two to three years. I would like the world to know that this is okay, normal, expected. I would like the world to know that my grief journey is about remembering my loved one, not trying to come to the point where I've pushed him out of my mind, or to the point where I've pushed him out of existence. My loved one lived, and his existence didn't end just because his physical life is over. I loved my husband, so please allow me to continue to express my love for him by allowing and expecting me to grieve.

*

GRACE YOUNG
Grace's son Jack died
in 2007 on his 27th birthday

It is my sincere wish that NO family lose a child to suicide for lack of understanding the ups and downs of depression. It is our hope that our annual music festival will lead those who are struggling to the proper avenues of help. I know that my son is safe in the arms of God, and that his life had purpose and meaning. I think he would be pleased that so many others have been saved, and have received the gift of life from Particle Accelerator, in memory of Jack Young Jr.

*

Be like the birds, sing after every storm.
-BETH MENDE CONNY

*

CHAPTER TWENTY

FINDING THE SUNRISE

One night in my own journey, I had one of *those* dreams: a vivid nightmare that stays with you. I was running westward in a frantic attempt to catch the setting sun as it descended below the horizon. Rapidly advancing from behind was nightfall; foreboding and frightening, it was a pitch black abyss. And it was coming directly for me. I ran as fast as my legs could go toward the sunset, but my attempt was futile; the sun descended below the horizon, out of my reach. Oh, the looming nightfall was terrifying! But it was clear that if I wanted to ever see the sun again, I had to stop running west and instead turn around and walk east to begin my journey through the great murky abyss . . . the nightfall of grief. For just as there would be no rainbow without the rain, the sun only rises on the other side of night.

The message was clear: it was futile to avoid my grief; I had to allow it to swallow me whole. Then, and only then, would I find my way through it and out the other side.

I remember reading in a bereavement book that if we don't allow ourselves to experience the full scope of the journey, it will come back to bite us. I couldn't fathom how it could get any worse, but I knew I didn't want to test that theory. So I gave in and allowed my grief to swallow me whole. I allowed myself to wail on my daughter's bedroom floor. I penned my deep emotions, regardless of who might read it. I created a national radio show to openly and candidly discuss our journeys with anyone who wanted to call in. And I allowed myself to sink to the bottom of the fiery pits of hell. This, in turn, lit a fire under me, so to speak, to find a way out.

Today, I'm often asked how I manage my grief so well. Some assume that because I have found peace and joy, I'm simply avoiding my grief. Others believe that because I work in the bereavement field, I'm wallowing in self-pity. Well, which is it?

Neither. I will miss my child with every breath I take. Just like you, I will always have my moments: the painful holidays, birthdays, death anniversaries, a song or smell that evokes an unexpected memory. But I have also found purpose, beauty and joy again. It takes hard work and determination to overcome profound grief, and it also takes the ability to let go and succumb to the journey. Do not be afraid of the tears, sorrow, and heartbreak; they are a natural reaction, and are imperative to your healing.

As you walk your own path, avail yourself to whatever bereavement tools that might ease your discomfort, for each one was created by someone who walked in your shoes and understands the heartache. While there are many wonderful bereavement resources available, what brings comfort to one person might irritate the next. Bereavement tools are not one-size-fits-all, so if one tool doesn't work, find another.

Lastly, grief is not something we get "over," like a mountain. Rather, it is something we get "through," like the rapids of Niagara Falls. Without the kayak and paddle. And plenty of falls. But it's also survivable. And if others had survived this wretched journey, why not me? And why not you? On the following pages are the baby steps I took to put hell in my rearview mirror. They took great effort at first, and lots of patience with myself. But like any dedicated routine, it got easier over time, and the reward of finding balance in my life was worth every step.

1. VALIDATING OUR EMOTIONS

The first step is to validate your emotions. When we talk about our deep heartbreak, we aren't ruminating in our sorrow or feeling sorry for ourselves. By discussing it, we are actually processing it. If we aren't allowed to process it, then it becomes silent grief. Silent grief is deadly grief.

Find a friend who will patiently listen while you discuss your loss for fifteen minutes every day. Set the timer, and ask them not to say anything during those fifteen minutes. Explain that it is important for you to just ramble without interruption, guidance, or judgment. You need not have the same listener each time, but practice this step every day.

2. COMPASSIONATE THOUGHTS

Find yourself a quiet spot. It can be your favorite chair, in your car, in your office, or even in your garden. Then clear your head and for five minutes think nothing but compassionate thoughts about yourself. Not your spouse, not your children, not your coworkers, but yourself. Having trouble? Fill in the blanks below, and then give yourself permission to really validate those positive qualities. Do this every day.

I have a _____

Example: good heart, gentle soul, witty personality

I make a _____

Example: good lasagna, potato salad, scrapbook, quilt

I'm a good_____

Example: friend, gardener, knitter, painter, poem writer

People would say I'm _____

Example: funny, kind, smart, gentle, generous, humble, creative

3. TENDER LOVING CARE

While grieving, it is important to consider yourself in the intensive care unit of Grief United Hospital, and treat accordingly. How would nurses treat you if you were their patient in the ICU? They would be compassionate, gentle, and allow for plenty of rest. That is exactly how you should treat yourself. Also, consider soothing your physical self with TLC as an attentive way to honor your emotional pain. This doesn't mean you have to book an expensive massage. If wearing fuzzy blue socks offers a smidgen of comfort, then wear them unabashedly. If whipped cream on your cocoa offers a morsel of pleasure, then indulge unapologetically.

Treating our five senses to anything that offers a perception of delight might not erase the emotional heartache, but it will offer a reminder that not all pleasure is lost. List five ways you can offer yourself tender loving care, and then incorporate <u>at least three</u> into your day, every day. With practice, the awareness of delight eventually becomes effortless, and is an important step toward regaining joy. TLC suggestions:

- Shower or bathe with a lovely scented soap
- Soak in a warm tub with Epsom salts or a splash of bath oil
- Wear a pair of extra soft socks
- Light a fragrant candle
- Listen to relaxing music
- Apply a rich lotion to your skin before bed
- Indulge in a few bites of your favorite treat
- Enjoy a mug of your favorite soothing herbal tea
- Add whipped cream to a steaming mug of cocoa
- _____
- _____

4. SEE THE BEAUTY

Listening to the birds outside my bedroom window every morning was something I had loved since childhood. But when Aly died, I found myself deaf and blind to the beauty around me. My world had become colorless and silent. On one particular morning as I struggled to get out of bed, I halfheartedly noticed the birds chirping outside my bedroom window. My heart sank as I realized that they had been chirping all along, but I was now deaf to their morning melody. Panic set in as I concluded that I would never enjoy life's beauty ever again. Briefly entertaining suicide to escape the profound pain, I quickly ruled it out. My family had been through so much already, I couldn't dump further pain on them. But in order to survive the heartbreak, I had to find a way to allow beauty back into my life.

So on that particular morning as I lay in bed, I forced myself to listen and really *hear* the birds. Every morning from that point forward, I repeated that same exercise. With persistent practice, it became easier and then eventually effortless to appreciate the birds' chirping and singsongs. Glorious beauty and sounds have once again returned to my world.

Profound grief can appear to rob our world of all beauty. Yet the truth is, and despite our suffering, beauty continues to surround us. The birds continue to sing, flowers continue to bloom, the surf continues to ebb and flow. Reconnecting to our surroundings helps us to reintegrate back into our environment.

Begin by acknowledging one small pleasantry each day. Perhaps your ears register the sound of singing birds. Or you catch the faint scent of warm cookies as you walk past a bakery. Or notice the sun's illumination of a nearby red rosebush. Give yourself permission to notice one pleasantry, and allow it to *really* register.

Here are some suggestions:

- Listen to the birds sing (hearing)
- Observe pretty cloud formations (sight)
- Visit a nearby park and listen to the children (hearing)
- Notice the pretty colors of blooming flowers (sight)
- Light a fragrant candle (scent)
- See the beauty in the sunset (sight)
- Attend a local recital, concert, play, or comedy act (hearing)
- Wear luxury socks (touch)
- Wrap yourself in a soft scarf or sweater (touch)
- Indulge in whipped cream on your cocoa (taste)
- Enjoy a Hershey's chocolate kiss (taste)

5. PROTECT YOUR HEALTH

After our daughter's accident I soon found myself fighting an assortment of viruses including head colds, stomach flus, sore throats and more, compounding my already frazzled emotions. Studies show that profound grief throws our body into "flight or fight" syndrome for months and months, which is very hard on our physical body. Thus, it becomes critical to guard our physical health. Incorporating a few changes into our daily routine feels hard at first, but soon gets easy. Plus, a stronger physical health helps to strengthen our coping skills. Below are a few suggestions to consider adding to your daily routine to help your physical self withstand the emotional upheaval.

- Practice good sleep hygiene
- Drink plenty of water
- Take a short walk outside every day
- Resist simple carbohydrates (I'm a food addict, so I know that avoiding simple carbs is worth its weight in gold)
- Keep a light calendar and guard your time carefully, don't allow others to dictate and overflow your schedule

6. FIND AN OUTLET

For a long time in the grief journey, everything is painful. In the early days, just getting out of bed and taking a shower can be exhausting. Housecleaning, grocery shopping, and routine errands often take a backseat or disappear altogether. As painful as it is, it's very important to find an outlet that gets you out of bed each day. Finding something to distract you from the pain, occupy your mind, and soothe your senses can be tricky, but possible. Performing a repetitive action can calm your mood, and even result in a new craft or gifts to give.

Beginning a new outlet may feel exhausting at first, just remember that the first step is always the hardest. And you don't have to do it forever, just focus on it for the time being.

Possible activities include:

- Learn to mold chocolate or make soap
- Learn how to bead, knit, crochet, or quilt
- Volunteer at a local shelter
- Learn a new sport such as golf or kayaking
- Create a memorial garden in a forgotten part of the yard
- Join Pinterest or a book club
- Doodle or draw
- Mold clay
- Learn to scrapbook
- Join a book club

Grief is hell on earth. It truly is. But when walking through hell, your only option is to keep going. Eventually the hell ends, the dark night fades to dawn, and the sun begins its ascent once again.

Just keep going and you, too, will find the sunrise.

Lynda Cheldelin Fell

My great hope is to laugh as much as I cry;
to get my work done and
try to love somebody and
have the courage to accept the love in return.
MAYA ANGELOU

*

MEET THE WRITERS

*

KAYLA ARNOLD

Kayla's uncle Tim died in 2001 at age 34

kayla_n_arnold@yahoo.com

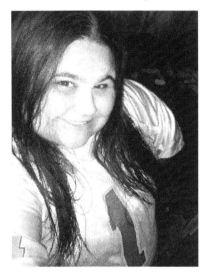 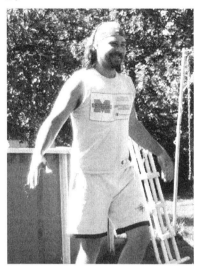

Kayla Nicholle Arnold was born near Santa Maria, California, at Vandenberg Air Force Base, and now lives in Battle Creek, Michigan. She has a great family and two younger sisters. Kayla has her associate degree in Nursing from Kellogg Community College. She is a diehard University of Michigan fan, a passion she learned from her Uncle Tim. Kayla is very happy to share her experience with suicide, and always loves it when she has the opportunity to help others understand and live with the pain we are left with from being a loved one left behind.

*

EMILY BARNHARDT

Emily's friend and roommate Hannah died in 2014 at age 20

changethatlasts90@gmail.com http://changethatlasts.weebly.com

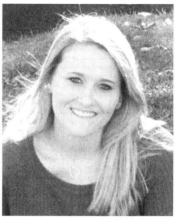

Emily Barnhardt was born and raised in Charlotte, North Carolina, where she lived with her parents and two siblings until age sixteen. She then attended boarding school in Asheville, North Carolina, for the remainder of high school. Emily began her undergraduate studies at the University of Denver in Colorado, dual-majoring in Business and in Hospitality Management. After her first two years of college, Emily endured many challenging circumstances in her personal life, and relocated to Boca Raton, Florida, at the age of twenty-two. Through the trials she experienced in life, Emily developed deep concern and empathy for people who were hurting, and realized her calling in life is helping others. She returned to

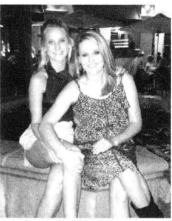

college at Florida Atlantic University to pursue a Master's degree in Social Work. She was awarded the AlyBlue Media Humanitarian Award 2015 for her extraordinary contribution to raising suicide awareness at such a young age. Emily finds strength, freedom, and restoration in her Christian faith, and contributes the healing and change in her life to the Lord. One year after her loss, she decided to move back home to Charlotte. She is currently working and continuing her degree in social work.

*

CHRISTINE BASTONE
Christine's sister Elizabeth died in 2012 at age 38
C.Bastone@mail.com   *   www.facebook.com/CricketsPlace1

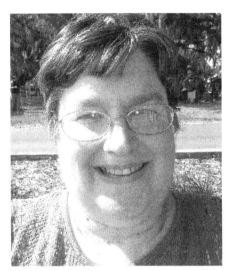
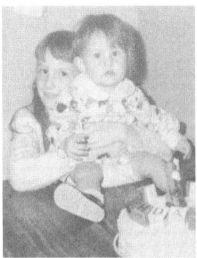

Christine Bastone is a stay-at-home mom in her forties who has only recently figured out that she wants to be a writer when she grows up! She was born in northeast Ohio and moved to Florida in May 1995. She married Angelo Bastone in July 1997. They have a son, Joshua, born in 2001, and a daughter, Katelyn, born in 2004. The four of them live at the end of a quiet street in central Florida. Christine has always loved to read, and was thrilled when her husband gave her a Kindle for Christmas in 2011. She has since read hundreds of Kindle books. Christine is co-author of *Grief Diaries: Loss of a Sibling*, and contributed to the book, *Faces of Suicide, Volume 1*, available on Amazon as a Kindle book. She has also been a guest on Grief Diaries Radio twice in 2014, both episodes are available on iTunes. At the time of this publication she is working on a new book called *Advice from Tomorrow*.

*

SHARON EHLERS
Sharon's best friend Joy died in 2009 at age 52
Sharon's former fiancé John died in 2012 at age 59
sharon@grief-reiki.com   *   www.grief-reiki.com

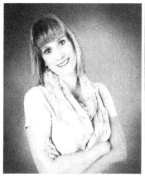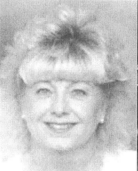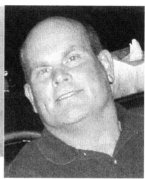

Sharon (Skura) Ehlers was born and raised in Los Angeles, California. She is most passionate about her three beautiful children, ages thirty-three, twenty-three, and twenty-one. She has loving parents and a beautiful sister who also live in Los Angeles. After the suicides of a close friend and a former fiancé within a two-year period, Sharon was confused about how many people either avoided her or didn't want to talk about these events. In her grief, she tried to make sense of it all, but it seemed like it was "never the right time" to bring it up with anyone. So Sharon took a deep breath and tried to work through the grief on her own. Her thought was that there had to be a better way. So after working in corporate America for almost thirty years, Sharon decided to start her own company, Grief Reiki® LLC, to offer a multidimensional approach to grief through emotional recovery and spiritual healing. Now a certified grief recovery specialist® and co-author of Grief Diaries: Surviving Loss by Suicide, Sharon is helping others to heal and recover from grief by providing them with a safe, compassionate and healing environment for their journey. Her best lesson in life is: "Miracles do happen."

*

BONNIE FORSHEY
Bonnie's son Billy died in 1993 at age 16
bonnieforshey@msn.com

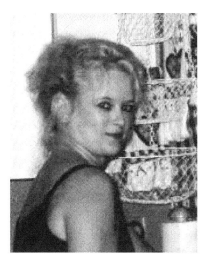 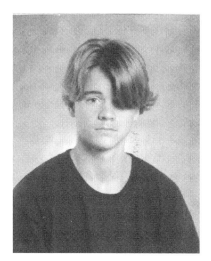

Bonnie Forshey was born in Lewistown, Pennsylvania, and raised in New Castle, Delaware. She later moved to Swainsboro, Georgia, where she attended Emanuel County Junior College. She earned a Science Merit Award and graduated with an A.S. degree. Later she attended Gordon State College in Barnesville, Georgia, earning a B.S. in Nursing.

She spent most of her life working in medical-surgical, geriatrics, rehabilitation and long-term care facilities. Bonnie also raised two children, and worked as a nursing assistant, unit secretary, and in medical records while putting herself through school. Bonnie has two grandsons and currently resides in both Port Royal, Pennsylvania, and Brandon, Florida.

*

LAURA HABEDANK
Laura's brother Brian died in 2010 at age 35
letterstobrianblog@yahoo.com * www.letterstobrianblog.com

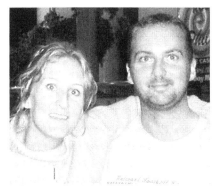 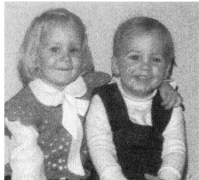

Laura Habedank is a Minnesota native but has called Austin, Texas, home since November 2009. She works in accounting for a large printing firm, where she has been employed since relocating to Texas.

In her spare time, she enjoys playing piano, singing, songwriting, and the occasional hike on the lovely greenbelt trails of Austin. She has an affinity for all things strange and, even at age forty-two, still finds whoopee cushions endlessly hilarious. She regularly consumes mass quantities of pizza and doughnuts while binge-watching the TV series *Six Feet Under* on her couch in the company of her two geriatric cats, Bear and Bubba. In the paraphrased words of the immortal Ron Burgundy of the Channel 4 news team, "She's kind of a big deal."

*

VICKI HECKROTH
Vicki's son Matthew died in 2000 at age 17

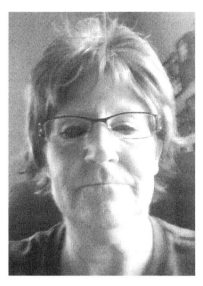 Vicki Heckroth was born in Spencer, Iowa, the second child of Bonnie and Gail Handy. She was welcomed at home by her older sister Terrie, and her brother Rodney was born three years later. Vicki spent her early years in Worthington, Minnesota, before moving to Greenville, Iowa, at age ten. Vicki was raised by her father and stepmother Shirley. She also had two halfsiblings, Kristi and Brian.

Vicki has been through a lot in life, beginning from the tender age of five, when her mom died in an automobile accident. She has weathered two very abusive relationships, having a granddaughter born with some issues and losing her youngest child and only son, 17-year-old Matthew, in 2000 to suicide.

Vicki is disabled from rheumatoid arthritis and several other health issues, though she was healthy until her son passed away. She has been married for twenty-five years, and has two daughters, thirty-five year-old Heidi and thirty-three year-old Melissa. She resides in Iowa, where she breeds Chihuahuas.

*

MARLISE MAGNA
Marlise's fiancé Blaine died in 2010 at age 36

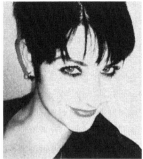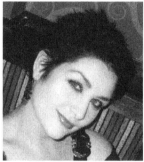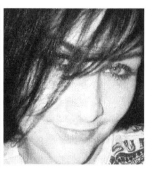

Marlise was born December 2, 1978, in Johannesburg, South Africa and is the oldest of two children. Her life has been nothing out of the ordinary, as most people would describe it. She studied drama at South Africa's National School of the Arts before becoming a Jill of all trades. She has worked as a canine behaviorist, wedding planner, TV presenter, matchmaker, and dance instructor, to name a few. At age thirty-five, after two divorces and many suicide attempts, she finally found what she wanted to do and is currently studying to become a pastor. She has been instrumental in planning two churches involved in relationship counseling, praise and worship singing. She is also lead singer in her own Christian band.

Marlise is also director of an alternative clothing and interior design company, magazine editor, and proofreader. Marlise is an avid reader and loves nothing better than performing research and playing trivia games. Standup comedy and watching reality TV series are also favorite pastime. She lives with her mom and her beloved dog, Juke.

*

MARCELLA MALONE

Marcella's brother Michael died in 2014 at age 20

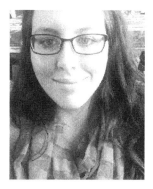 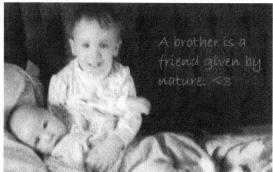

Marcella Malone was born and raised in Marshall, Michigan. She was a middle child between two boys, Timothy, who eight years older, and Michael, who was one year younger. Growing up, she loved the outdoors, sports, and agriculture-related activities.

Marcella is the mother of a beautiful one-year-old boy. She is currently working as a home health aide while attending Wayne State University to obtain her B.S. in Psychology. Following graduation in May, she plans to continue her education to receive her Master's in Social Work.

*

JULIE MJELVE
Julie's husband Cameron died in 2011 at age 42
julie@grievingtogether.ca   *   www.grievingtogether.ca

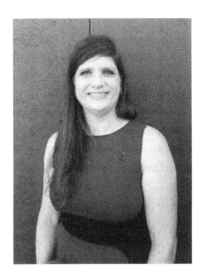 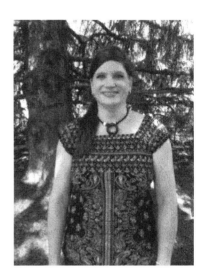

Julie (McCargar) Mjelve was born in Edmonton, Alberta, Canada. She completed her BSC in Physical Therapy in 1992. After working as a physical therapist for ten years, Julie spent almost eight months traveling Europe before returning to Edmonton to complete her Master's in Education, specializing in teaching English as a Second Language. In 2007 Julie married James Cameron Mjelve. They went on to have three beautiful children - one boy and two girls. As the demands of child raising increased, Julie's work shifted from teaching English as a second language to internationally educated nurses to working as an academic strategist with a local college. Following the birth of their second child, Julie became a stay-at-home mom, focusing on the care and attention her children required. Currently, Julie has started her own business, along with two other partners, called Grieving Together which provides mourning symbols to those who are grieving.

*

BRIDGET PARK
Bridget's brother Austin died in 2008 at age 14
www.bridgetpark.com

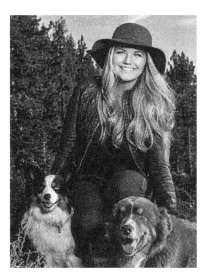 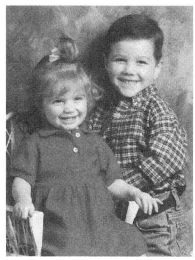

Bridget Park was born and raised on a cattle and sheep ranch in northern Nevada. She lost her older brother Austin in 2008 to suicide. Since then she has learned to make the best out of this tragedy and to honor her brother by writing and publishing *Growing Young: A Memoir of Grief*.

Bridget is currently twenty years old and a student at Oklahoma State University. While being a full-time student, she engages in speaking engagements around the country.

*

GRACE YOUNG
Grace's son Jack died in 2007 on his 27th birthday
www.particleaccelerator.org

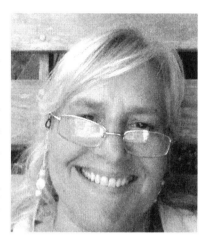

Grace Lannon Young fell in love with Jack Young Sr. in 1976 while she was still in high school. They were married in 1979 in Putnam, Connecticut. Grace loved being a mother to Jack Jr., born in 1980, and to Benjamin in 1981. They bought a house a few blocks from Grace's mom, and took great joy in raising their two precious sons. They worshiped God together at the local Baptist church, and loved to sing together while Grace played the guitar or piano. Grace loved to play music and also loved to draw and write poetry, skills that both of her children emulated well. Grace enjoyed gardening, walking, and playing outside with the children, and often had more than one of her friends' children in her charge. She was fortunate enough to be a stay-

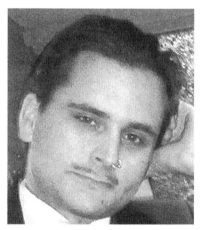

at-home mother until the kids went to school. She worked as a secretary for many years at the local hospital, and after a lengthy recuperation from a back injury and surgery, went back to work at a plumbing supply house. Grace now devotes her time to caring for her elderly mom and her three grandsons, and increasing awareness of suicide and depression through Particle Accelerator.

THANK YOU

I am deeply indebted to the writers who contributed to *Grief Diaries: Surviving Loss by Suicide*. It required a tremendous amount of courage to revisit such painful memories for the purpose of helping others, and the collective dedication to seeing the project to the end is a legacy to be proud of.

I appreciate author Annah Elizabeth's assistance in framing the start of each chapter. I'm also grateful to our Grief Diaries village and the very lovely souls I consider dear friends, collaborative partners, mentors, and muses. I treasure each and every one of you!

There simply are no words to express how much I love my husband Jamie, our children, and our wonderfully supportive family and friends for being there through laughter and tears, and encouraging me at every turn. None of this would have been possible without their unquestioning love that continues to surround me.

Finally, I am indebted to our daughter Aly for being my biggest cheerleader in Heaven. Her bright star continues to inspire me, and I can feel her love through the thin veil that separates us as I work to offer help, healing and hope around the world. My dearest Lovey, I love you to the fartherest star and beyond. XO

Lynda Cheldelin Fell

Shared joy is doubled joy;
shared sorrow is half a sorrow.
SWEDISH PROVERB

*

ABOUT

LYNDA CHELDELIN FELL

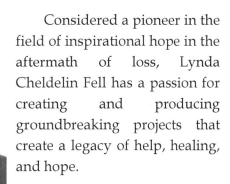

Considered a pioneer in the field of inspirational hope in the aftermath of loss, Lynda Cheldelin Fell has a passion for creating and producing groundbreaking projects that create a legacy of help, healing, and hope.

She is the creator of the 5-star book series *Grief Diaries*, board president of the National Grief & Hope Coalition, and CEO of AlyBlue Media. Her repertoire of interviews include Dr. Martin Luther King's daughter, Trayvon Martin's mother, sisters of the late Nicole Brown Simpson, Pastor Todd Burpo of Heaven Is For Real, CNN commentator Dr. Ken Druck, and other societal newsmakers on finding healing and hope in the aftermath of life's harshest challenges.

Lynda's own story began in 2007, when she had an alarming dream about her young teenage daughter, Aly. In the dream, Aly was a backseat passenger in a car that veered off the road and landed in a lake. Aly sank with the car, leaving behind an open book floating face down on the water. Two years later, Lynda's dream became reality when her daughter was killed as a backseat passenger in a car accident while coming home from a swim meet.

Overcome with grief, Lynda's forty-six-year-old husband suffered a major stroke that left him with severe disabilities, changing the family dynamics once again.

The following year, Lynda was invited to share her remarkable story about finding hope after loss, and she accepted. That cathartic experience inspired her to create ground-breaking projects spanning national events, radio, film and books to help others who share the same journey feel less alone. Now an award-winning and international bestselling author, Lynda is dedicated to helping ordinary people share their own extraordinary stories.

Because of that floating book her daughter left behind, Lynda understands that the dream she had in 2007 was actually a glimpse into a divine plan destined to bring comfort, healing and hope to people around the world.

lynda@lyndafell.com | www.lyndafell.com | www.griefdiaries.com

GRIEF DIARIES

ABOUT THE SERIES

It's important that we share our experiences with other people. Your story will heal you, and your story will heal somebody else. -IYANLA VANZANT

Grief Diaries is a ground-breaking series of anthology books featuring true stories about real life experiences. The collection of stories highlights the spirit of human resiliency, explores intimate aspects of each experience, and offers comfort and hope to those who share the same path. The series began with eight books exploring losses shared by people around the world. Over a hundred people in six countries registered, and the books were launched in December 2015. Now home to more than 450 writers spanning the globe, Grief Diaries has 17 titles in print with 13 more due by the end of 2016. Another 20 titles are set to be added in 2017.

Now a 5-star series, a portion of profits from every book in the series goes to national organizations serving those in need.

Humanity's legacy of stories and storytelling is the most precious we have.
All wisdom is in our stories and songs.
DORIS LESSING

*

ALYBLUE MEDIA TITLES

PUBLISHED

Grief Diaries: Surviving Loss of a Spouse

Grief Diaries: Surviving Loss of a Child

Grief Diaries: Surviving Loss of a Sibling

Grief Diaries: Surviving Loss of a Parent

Grief Diaries: Surviving Loss of an Infant

Grief Diaries: Surviving Loss of a Loved One

Grief Diaries: Surviving Loss by Suicide

Grief Diaries: Surviving Loss of Health

Grief Diaries: How to Help the Newly Bereaved

Grief Diaries: Loss by Impaired Driving

Grief Diaries: Through the Eyes of an Eating Disorder

Grief Diaries: Loss by Homicide

Grief Diaries: Loss of a Pregnancy

Grief Diaries: Living with a Brain Injury

Grief Diaries: Hello from Heaven

Grief Diaries: Grieving for the Living

Grief Diaries: Shattered

Grief Diaries: Project Cold Case

Grief Diaries: Through the Eyes of Men

Grammy Visits From Heaven

Faith, Grief & Pass the Chocolate Pudding

FORTHCOMING TITLES (PARTIAL LIST):

Heaven Talks to Children

Color My Soul Whole

Grief Reiki

Grief Diaries: Through the Eyes of a Funeral Director

Grief Diaries: You're Newly Bereaved, Now What?

Grief Diaries: Life After Organ Transplant

Grief Diaries: Raising a Disabled Child

Grief Diaries: Through the Eyes of Cancer

Grief Diaries: Poetry & Prose and More

Grief Diaries Life After Rape

Grief Diaries: Living with Mental Illness

There's a bright future for you at every turn,
even if you miss one.

*

To share your story in a Grief Diaries book,
visit www.griefdiaries.com

PUBLISHED BY ALYBLUE MEDIA
Inside every human is a story worth sharing.
www.AlyBlueMedia.com

Printed in Great Britain
by Amazon

REVIVING DEMOCRACY

CITIZENS AT THE HEART OF GOVERNANCE

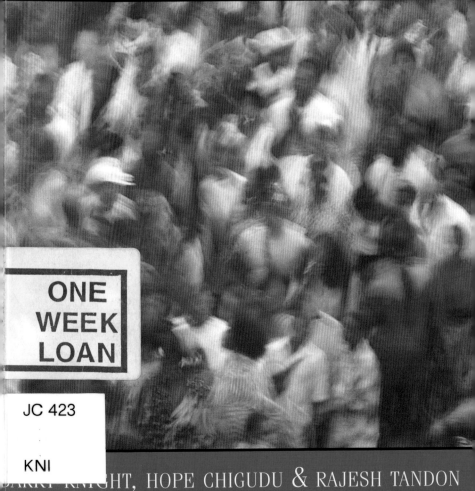

BARRY KNIGHT, HOPE CHIGUDU & RAJESH TANDON

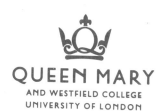

QUEEN MARY
AND WESTFIELD COLLEGE
UNIVERSITY OF LONDON

THE LIBRARY

JC 423 KN1

Reviving Democracy